MAKING SENSE OF THE
CORONAVIRUS
PANDEMIC OF
2020

Richard Henry
M.D.

QUEEN'S UNIVERSITY
Kingston, Ontario, Canada

MAKING SENSE OF THE CORONAVIRUS PANDEMIC OF 2020

Beverley Street Books
80 Beverley Street, Kingston, Ontario
www.beverleystreet.com

Cover design by: Lynne McMullan

Library and Archives Canada Cataloging in Publication information is available upon request

ISBN 978-1-7771290-1-9

DEDICATION

This book is dedicated to the memory of

Dr. Li Wenliang
(12 October 1986 – 7 February 2020)

In December of 2019, Dr. Li Wenliang, aged 33, was working as an Ophthalmologist at Wuhan Central Hospital when he was made aware that patients in his hospital appeared to be infected with a new coronavirus. He shared this information in a private social media chat group. As happens with social media, screenshots of his messages went viral and he was cautioned by his hospital's Supervision Department. The Wuhan Police Department followed also issued him with a formal warning for "making false comments on the internet."

Dr. Wenliang continued working at the hospital under the pall of a reprimand. On January 7 2020 he contracted the virus himself. Three days later he developed a fever and cough and was admitted under quarantine to the hospital where he worked. He finally tested positive on January 30 2020, three weeks after he was admitted.

On February 4, the Chinese People's Court ruled that the Covid-19 whistleblowers, including Dr. Wenliang, should not have been criticized for their outspokenness. Dr. Wenliang felt relief that the top court had not only exonerated him but also criticized the police's actions. These were probably his last words on the subject:

"I think there should be more that one voice in a healthy society, and I don't approve of using public power for excessive interference."

On February 5 2020 Dr. Wenliang started to feel short of breath and his oxygen saturation dropped to 85%. His heart stopped later that night.

Dr. Wenliang is survived by his wife and their two children.

Sourced from Dr. Wenliang's obituary
published in *The Lancet*, February 29 2020, Volume 395, page 682.

FOREWORD

A First-hand Account of the SARS Epidemic in 2003

"I was working in Hong Kong as an anesthesiologist at the Prince of Wales Hospital (PWH) when the outbreak of the SARS epidemic occurred. The first hint of trouble came in December 2002 with the news that there was a shortage of *vinegar* in Guangdong province, just across the border in Mainland China as people there were using it as a disinfectant. A flu-like illness was going around and it seemed to be spreading fast and making people very ill.

The new illness came to us on February 21 2003, when a physician who had been treating patients with the disease in Guangzhou, the capital city of Guangdong province, travelled to Hong Kong and booked into the Metropole Hotel. The following day he sought help at a public hospital, where he was admitted with respiratory distress and later died from his illness.

Seven hotel guests on the same floor in the Metropole Hotel unknowingly contracted the virus from the doctor. Six of them flew back to their respective countries: Singapore (3), Vietnam (1) and Canada (2). That was how the virus spread around the world. The seventh person was a local man who was admitted to my hospital, PWH, on March 4. He was the first person to introduce the virus to PWH.

Later that same month, a 33-year old man from Shenzhen city in Guangdong province in Mainland China visited Hong Kong. He attended PWH as an outpatient for kidney dialysis while staying with his brother in a high-rise apartment housing estate called Amoy Gardens. The young man subsequently developed diarrhea and was admitted to PWH. His brother, sister-in-law and 2 nurses who looked after him in hospital later became ill. The virus also spread at Amoy Gardens and went on to infect 329 people, killing 33.

The virus likely spread through contact with the elevator buttons and possibly the sewage system in the buildings. Hong Kong plumbing has a peculiar system of drainage from the bathroom floors through a U-trap drainpipe that must be filled with water to prevent exhaust of sewer gas from the pipes. I recall smelling sewage in my apartment after someone on the floors above me flushed their toilet when my U-trap was not properly filled with water. I still wonder if there were enough viruses in that sewer gas to spread the infection.

The Amoy Garden outbreak in March marked the peak of the SARS epidemic in Hong Kong. Although a second, smaller peak occurred in mid-April, it petered out by June. All told, there were 1755 documented SARS cases in Hong Kong, with 299 deaths (17%). Eight of the 386 healthcare workers who were infected, 4 doctors, 1 nurse and 3 healthcare assistants, died.

PWH was at the epicenter of the infection because it was contaminated early in the outbreak and was made a designated SARS hospital. Over 100 of our hospital staff were infected. My Anesthesiology Department was at the forefront of the battle. Elective surgeries were cancelled and critically ill patients who did not have SARS were transferred to other hospitals. Those of us in direct contact with SARS patients were quarantined in a designated apartment building about twenty minutes walk from the hospital. We were not allowed to go home to our families until the outbreak was over.

We resorted to treating SARS patients with the antiviral drug ribavirin and steroids to reduce lung inflammation, using large doses of steroids in severely ill patients until they either recovered or died. Many of those desperately ill patients did die. A local doctor who we were treating had contracted SARS while visiting his daughter, herself a medical student hospitalized with the infection. After treatment with high dose steroids he ruptured his bowel and required emergency surgery. I was assigned to be his anesthesiologist.

Before the surgery started I sent my resident home, as there was no need for both of us to get infected. We operated in an isolation room with negative pressure airflow instead of the usual positive pressure operating rooms. We switched the usual surgery facemasks to 3M *AirMate* facemasks to try to protect ourselves. Upon opening the peritoneal cavity, there was so much feces in the abdomen that it gushed out and poured onto the floor. Inflammation was causing fluid accumulation in his lungs that I was barely able to get enough oxygen into him. Surgery went on for four hours before I could take him back to the intensive care unit, where he spent another two weeks fighting for his life and I am happy to say, survived. His daughter made a much easier recovery.

I think this may have been the only SARS patient who required surgery during that epidemic. We now know that using large, desperate doses of steroids for a prolonged period was not helpful and likely made things worse. Bowel perforation is just one of those complications.

During SARS, our whole Hong Kong society and its healthcare systems were severely challenged. That was also when I saw the best of humanity. While in quarantine, we received donated food and fruits from the public in appreciation. During the funeral of some of the healthcare workers who had succumbed to the virus, people lined the streets to show their respect. The hospitals and their staff, the government, and the general public responded responsibly and efficiently to bring the crisis to an end.

With Covid-19, I am seeing my hospital colleagues springing into action. I knew all along that they were excellent doctors, nurses, support staff, and administrators. Now I also see that they are superb organizers, innovators, and selfless individuals. Together, I know we can all get through this."

Dr. Anthony Ho
Professor, Department of Anesthesiology
and Peri-operative Medicine
QUEEN'S UNIVERSITY
Kingston, Ontario, Canada

Umuntu Ngumuntu Ngabantu

'I am because you are, and you are because we are.'

'*Ubuntu*' is the essence of African Humanism – 'that which cultivates a sense of self-worth by esteeming the inner being of a person as a full and valued member of their community, integrating *person* to *people*.'

The spirit of Ubuntu is deeply rooted in the Xhosa and Zulu nations of South Africa and is personified by Nelson Mandela.

The pressing need to observe this powerful message of collective action could not be timelier. Covid-19 will test us in many ways, individually and as communities.

❀

CONTENTS

CONTENTS

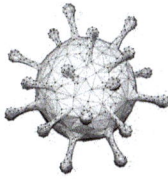

PROLOGUE

Exhortation: One Virus to Another.

I wrote this little story as an allegorical synopsis of CoV2. My friends enjoyed it, so I have included it.

A bat-borne virus sends his cloned offspring into the world, wanting for his scion what every virus would want for himself.

"Son, the time has come for us to go our separate ways. Before you leave, I am going to tell you what you must do to become a formidable conqueror.

It is time for you to forego this life amongst bats. We have infected them for thousands of years and they know us too well. They make life hard for us. We need a new host species, one that has no knowledge of our ways, and is not always expecting us with handcuffs ready to prevent us from entering their cells. I have decided that you must start infecting humans.

From this very place we are in now, humans will soon start spreading out in vast numbers all over China to celebrate their New Year with their families. Humans travel incessantly and with great speed. Because of their habits, you will reach every outpost of their existence before they even feel you. You will see the world. Wherever you find them living closely together you will spread amongst them with ease, faster than even I could hope for you. You might infect hundreds of people in a matter of hours as you are exhaled by a single human at a music concert.

You have been given the perfect weapon, honed over thousands of iterations. The spikes on your envelope are the pride of our coronavirus heritage. Although your older brother used them well to spread in humans, in the end his efforts proved futile. I have worked hard and I think you are now ready.

As you spread between humans, you may find yourself in a small floating droplet of their lung fluid. This is the key to spreading yourself. When other humans breath, you will be inhaled deep into their lungs. You will know you are there because a protein called Ace2 will be waiting to greet you. As you embrace in our familiar viral greeting, a fearsome looking protein called Tempress will unzip the tight bonds of your protective envelope. Do not be afraid, but ignore it. If you let go of Ace2, Tempress will harm you.

After you are unzipped, be cautious and use your freedom to get even closer to Ace2. Ace2 will become alarmed and, in trying to defend itself, will cut your arms loose allowing you to grab onto the cell. In a third and last desperate attempt to stop you, Tempress will cut off the outer piece of Ace2, hoping to free it from your grasp. That is your cue to pull with your arms while you bite even harder. When Ace2 retreats to safety make it take you with it by holding on tightly. Other virus families have done this and it works well.

When you get inside the cell, shake off Ace2 and let your replication team go to work. My next instructions are critical, for your work is not yet done. This is what is going to bring you success. You must find the inner Ace2 on the nuclear membrane. The nucleus is where they keep all of their recipes to make their defensive weapons. Bind to nuclear Ace2 so that it shuts down the nucleus. CoV1 was unable to do this and humans detected his presence too soon.

Silencing the nucleus will allow you to begin cloning and start spreading without interference. Some humans will never know you have been there, even after you are fully replicated. Take as much time as you need. Try not to make mistakes when making copies of your code. It has taken a lot of work to get it right. I doubt you will be able to improve it.

When you leave the cell, hopefully your host will not have sounded the alarm by raising the temperature. Go on and infect as many cells as you can, sending clones down the rivers of fluid that circulate around their bodies. Many other cells will have Ace2 waiting to welcome you.

After you are shed, your spiked envelope will continue to serve you well. You will be able to stay alive for days; so don't panic if you don't get transmitted right away. You are designed to thrive in small groups. A few of you in a small aerosol droplet have an excellent chance of getting into the next human. If you land before you are breathed in, another human or animal will ingest you.

Things will start to get difficult as humans try to drive you off. Hang on for as long as you can. You can always hide in one of the animals they keep for their own use. If you end up in one of their pets, make the best of it. At this point, you will be on your own. You will not have a manual for this but you have my permission to change your code, beautiful as it is. Try different mutations. You might even find bits of animal code you can steal or their viruses may help you.

Later, if you find that humans have antibodies waiting for you, then you may alter your envelope so as not to be recognized. Do this gradually. Make small changes, just enough to blend in again, but not enough to prevent you from binding to Ace2 and enticing Tempress to unzip you.

As you change and adapt, always remember, it does not matter what happens to your hosts, or even what kind of animal they are. It is best not to alarm or even hurt them, as that will make them angry and they will try to kill you. Your mission is to infect as many humans as possible. All of these instructions are in your code, so protect it.

Those humans worthy of survival will find ways to cope with you. If *you* are worthy, you will become part of their existence. You will have freed us from the world of bats, before there are no bats left in the world. You will have a great future with humans as your hosts. You might even travel to other planets with them.

I have named you CoV2. I did this to honor your older brother, CoV1, who made a brave attempt to infect humans not too long ago. I have fixed his failings. Ace2 and Tempress will welcome you and help you to infect millions of humans.

Off you go now! Get to the nearest human. Snakes, civets and pangolins have helped us along the way in the past, or you may reach them on your own. It does not matter how you infect the first one."

❧ ❧ ❧

"I have brought myself, by long meditation,

to the conviction that a human being

with a settled purpose must accomplish it,

and that nothing can resist a will

which will stake even existence upon its fulfillment."

Benjamin Disraeli

❧

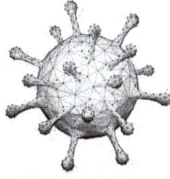

THE MAKINGS OF A PANDEMIC

Covid-19 is another chapter in the story about the ongoing interaction between viruses and life on earth. This viral pandemic is not our first, nor will it be our last. Spreading is what successful viruses do. It is in their DNA, or RNA. Our rising population density makes it so much easier for them.

Viruses are constantly changing. They do this inadvertently by making small mistakes, called mutations, when replicating themselves. Viral mutations are random and occur when viruses replicate themselves in their host cells. Coding missteps alter the proteins they make, which changes the way the proteins interact with their hosts, even making new host species susceptible. These random changes are called *genetic evolution*.

2019-CoV-2 is the novel beta coronavirus that is responsible for the Covid-19 pandemic of 2020. I have nicknamed it *CoV2*. It emerged in late 2019 with a novel gene sequence that altered the proteins in its outer envelope. Occasionally, when a random error is advantageous to the virus, it is called a *gain-of-function* mutation. When this does occur, the new virus outperforms its family members and a new strain is born.

Humans have changed, too, over the past few hundred years and especially the past fifty years. While we have *not* mutated our genes over that time, we have adopted a drastically different lifestyle. Although our genes dictate our innate abilities and are built into our genetic codes, we each have to activate those genes to enable those functions. You may come from a long line of weight lifters, marathon runners or swimmers, but you will not perform the same way without making the same effort.

Training, practicing and conditioning are all examples of *epigenetics* at work. When we make demands of our bodies, specific genes are activated to enable our bodies to meet those demands. We are continually adapting to our environment, and our lifestyles. Our bodies never stop responding to stress, even though our current stressors are very different from the 'forces of nature' that originally shaped us.

Since gravity prevents us from simply floating effortlessly, the genetic ability to make bones and muscles was honed over millions of years. Even so, exercise is still necessary to activate those same genes to maintain healthy bones and muscles in all of us.

Even though human genes have changed imperceptibly over thousands of years, we are very different from our ancestors. We are continually *changing our environment* and that alters how we *use* our genes. Our technological advances increasingly relieve us from arduous labor, weary walking, and frigid temperatures, blinding sunlight and gnawing hunger. Instead, many of us have adapted to eating and storing vast quantities of food as fat while we sit for most of our lives in comfortably thermo-neutral environments. These adaptations make us increasingly obese and barely able to run, hunt or live in the wild; yet, by our sheer numbers, we seem to be thriving. It's called *phenotypic evolution*.

Having turned our backs on our primordial history, our modern lifestyles may be putting us at risk from this new virus. True, the virus's mutations account for its increased ability to spread and our increased population density certainly helps; however, it does not explain why so many people dying after catching what some have dismissively called a 'cold'. What is peculiar about those who sicken and die, while others hardly even cough?

In this pandemic of 2020, a new viral *genotype* meets our modern human *phenotype*. Having made it this far, both viruses and humans are proven survivors. Once again, we are squaring off in another showdown.

CoV2 has been changing its genetic code, while we have been changing how we use ours.

If spread is a measure of the success of a virus then this one is a champion. Viral success does not depend on killing its host. The fact that only some of us die may have more to do with *us* than the virus. After all, we are all getting infected with the *same* virus. Human health, especially as we age, seems to be at the root of our different responses to an infection.

As this story is as much about human evolution as it is about viral mutations, we shall delve into the key human homeostatic system that is challenged the most to cope with the stresses of our modern lifestyle. Metabolic stress has become an exceedingly common part of the human condition and affects over half of the human population. Although we make valiant attempts to treat the diseases that result from this 'metabolic syndrome', our medical workarounds have not been very successful to date and may have put us directly in harms way from this newly emerged virus.

We shall also look at how viruses function, *making sense* of this particular virus and the changes responsible for its formidable gain-of-function. The virus has evolved to be an incredible spreader, no question, but it is likely our own relatively recent adaptations that have made us so susceptible to its effects.

As you go through this book you will understand how an everyday viral mutation that likely conferred little benefit while in its bat host, enabled CoV2 to infect a new mammalian species. There may have been an intermediate host species, or a laboratory, where further mutations perfected the virus for its debut in humans.

Once we understand how this virus impairs the very system that is trying to help us adapt to our new lifestyles, it will be easy to see how Covid-19 has the potential to challenge our individual survival.

The Collective Human Experience

We have all been thrust into this world, seemingly without our permission. We have all gasped for our first breath, cried for food and felt relief with each void of our bowels and bladders. And then we just kept right on going, increasing our interaction with our own micro-worlds each day. At its core, it's just biology. It just happened and keeps on happening. It is this collective experience that binds us physically and spiritually, even as we compete with each other for survival.

As 2020 gets underway, we are all in the path of another shared biological challenge that threatens our precarious equilibrium. As CoV2 *infects* many of us it will *affect* all of us. It is going to test our resilience and our intellects. Will it tear us apart or will it force us to build better societies with more stable and integrated lives? Each one of us will be asked to contribute as we merge with this virus.

If CoV2 continues to spread though our population, then we are going to have to embrace the challenge and work to get as many of us safely through the epidemic as possible. Today the official reports are 64,435 cases in 25 countries with 1383 deaths and just 2 deaths outside of China. These numbers may represent a 5% tip of the iceberg and the actual number of infected cases is likely 20 times greater already. By the time you read this book you might find these numbers nostalgically low.

Early in the outbreak of a new virus, it may be difficult to appreciate the virus's potential to both spread and cause disease. Already CoV2 looks a lot worse than its older siblings, SARS and MERS. I hope, after reading this book, you will be able to make sense of it all and be able to tackle it head-on, like a Springbok winning the 2019 World Cup of Rugby!

Knowledge and Action

Personal and collective knowledge provide the very essence of survival of a species. Some of this knowledge is *innate*, seemingly passed on in DNA, the inherited blueprints that each living creature carries. As summer comes to an end, geese know to fly south and squirrels know to start hiding food.

Acquired knowledge requires us to learn about our world, taking instructions from our parents and teachers at first. Later, we make personal decisions as to our best courses of action. We are an intelligent species and seem bent on building complex lives, even as some amongst us question the wisdom of this ever-increasing complexity.

We have flourished over the past few millennia and can presume that we have done a lot of things right, but challenges like this are an intermittent natural stress that will test our defenses. If we have strayed, we will pay the price. This could be one of those necessary corrective forces of nature that challenges our collective knowledge and highlights where modifications are needed.

Along with our scientific advances, we are still trying to integrate socially and economically by fostering healthy co-operation in place of destructive competition. We are making slow and painful gains towards breaking our inherited constructs of national and racial identity, seeking to replace them with something more inclusive and representative. Unfortunately, in the face of this threat, we may retreat back into our old paradigms in search of familiarity and safety.

Fear can be used as a strong motive to collectivize and enforce obedience. An inflexible approach is vulnerable to mistakes, and mistakes can be especially compounded when dissenting voices are eliminated. On the other hand, a collective that embraces self-reflection and tolerates new ideas can remain strong and viable. While working cohesively, we should be mindful of the last words of Dr. Wenliang and be careful to tolerate and promote individual thought.

This book is a narrative of a collection of relevant scientific knowledge that has already passed our collective scientific approval: peer-reviewed publication. True to the spirit of science, this narrative is my hypothesis of how I think the pieces of science fit together in this pandemic. All scientific knowledge should be shared and I share this hypothesis knowing that it will be scrutinized. I hope you enjoy understanding this aspect of the complexity of nature.

Why We Keep Having Outbreaks

New infectious diseases are constantly emerging in humans and animals, as evidenced by the 400 new infectious diseases identified since 1940. This emergence is a natural process that results from both increasing human interaction with animals and increasing human population densities.

Most of our established human infections originated in other animals. Viruses existed long before large animals and humans, so they must have been passed on between species that evolved before us. When a virus crosses into a new species, it is called a *zoonotic v*irus and it is said to cause a *zoonotic disease.* Most of our zoonotic viruses come from other *mammals* (80%) and birds. Sometimes an intermediary animal is used as a vector to bridge the gap between the original host and humans. Bat viruses can infect pangolins and camels, which in turn can infect humans. It's harder for viruses to cross from birds to mammals, which might explain why 'Bird flu' is not endemic in humans yet.

Equally, more than 50% of human pathogens can infect other animals, especially mammals. A virus can spread to other species and then animal-to-animal, even returning back to humans in an altered form with increased ability to harm us (pathogenicity). With 5000 known species of mammals and 10,000 species of birds, each with its own endemic virus populations, there are literally thousands of viruses waiting to be discovered.[1]

Pathogens are said to follow Tobler's First Law: '*near things are more related than distant things*'. Viruses and their hosts form interactive connected communities that are distinct and contained. However, increasing human contact with wild animals and our burgeoning global connectivity is tearing down the modularity that may have effectively isolated many viruses up till now.[2]

In 2009, the US Agency for International Development initiated the Emerging Pandemic Threats Program to predict and rapidly identify emerging zoonotic infections. They identify regions, wildlife hosts and human-animal interfaces that are likely to enable the next zoonotic emergence.

An arm of this program, known as 'PREDICT', operates in 20 developing countries with emerging infectious disease hotspots to identify likely human-animal interfaces. They collect samples in the field to identify new zoonotic viruses and new pathogenic mutations in known viruses. By 2013, they had collected 100,000 samples from 20,000 animals (bats, rodents, primates) in those 20 countries and discovered 150 new viruses. One wonders whether, in their altruistic attempt to build a defensive strategy, PREDICT could one day inadvertently become an intermediate zoonotic host themselves?[1]

There are three different types of community infectious events: emergence, outbreak and re-emergence. Emergence is the first record of an outbreak of a new virus in a given country. Emergence of a 'novel' virus, one that humans have never experienced before, requires time to fully comprehend. An outbreak is a recurrent event of something already experienced within the past 3 years and re-emergence is when an outbreak re-occurs after a period of 3 years.

If an emerging outbreak spreads, it becomes an epidemic. When it spreads around the world quickly it's a 'time-to panic epidemic', a pandemic. Pandemic potential is based on the number of people in a susceptible population who get infected by one infected person. A highly contagious virus infecting a new host population that has no previous immunity creates a pandemic scenario. A pandemic is especially concerning if the infection causes morbidity (sickness) and has an appreciable mortality (death) rate. Covid-19 is now officially a pandemic and is quickly proving to be the worst in living memory.

Limiting the Spread of Outbreaks

This pandemic of 2020 is going to test our individual and collective behavioral responses, especially as SARS, MERS, Swine flu, Bird flu, Ebola and Zika have already fatigued our emotional stress responses. Even my children were beyond tired of me warning about the inevitability of the next big-scary-viral-epidemic. I confess to resorting to a "Bird flu is coming" refrain to encourage my youngest daughter to finish her dinner a few too many times.

What we do when the threat becomes real, our behavioral responses, can be divided into three main silos.

Preventative behaviors: hand washing, protected coughing and sneezing, cleaning surfaces, wearing masks and vaccination. Not shaking hands and hugging one another is going to have to become, not just socially acceptable, but also respectful and the even the law.

Avoidance behaviors: personally avoiding crowds and public places, while governing bodies cancel events that draw crowds. Quarantining of infected individuals and groups can be self-imposed or mandated. Limiting travel, especially to of from heavily infected regions.

Management of disease: antiviral medicines, oxygenation/ventilation to minimize morbidity and death.

Adoptions of beneficial responses to a viral pandemic are known to vary between countries and cultures, and according to age, gender and education. Since fear of harm is a significant motivator for behavioral changes, the extent of motivation depends on both the severity and likelihood of harm. Converting that fear-driven motivation into action depends on our individual and collective ability to adopt harm-prevention strategies.

Each of us will assess our individual risk posed by Covid-19 and weigh that risk against our belief in the effectiveness of the actions required. We then weigh that assessment against our ability to put those actions into effect. In the end, what we each choose to do will reflect our overall perception of the threat. While a higher level of general anxiety increases the chance of us carrying out defensive behaviors, over reacting may result in behaviors that are more harmful to others and ourselves than the threat itself. An example of this would be overdosing on chloroquine in the hope of preventing Cov2 infection.

This is where things get tricky for governments. Motivating a population to adopt preventative and avoidant behavior may initially appear counterproductive, especially before the threat has materialized. If the measures are adopted early enough to be effective, the population might only perceive what was lost and be unable to appreciate what was avoided. Governments must encourage and enforce behavior that prevents spread, but more importantly, governments must do everything possible to *support appropriate behavior.*

Conversely, governments' failure to tell the whole story will result in a loss of trust, especially when threats start to materialize. People stop trusting when they are left feeling unprepared and a lack of political trust is highly detrimental to controlling a disease. In times of uncertainty, negative events that destroy trust are more noticeable than positive events. When people discredit risk assessments provided by authorities they are less likely to change behavior.

Communication and knowledge are important in preventing disease spread. The government of Singapore performed well during the SARS outbreak in 2004 and is still leading in trust in 2020. Since Singaporeans enjoy the benefits of their social collectivism, they are more obedient, no matter how strict or odious the regulations that are imposed on them.

The most important goal of all humanity in 2020 is, inarguably, to reduce the spread of CoV2. Our physical, social and economic health is at risk. You may be young and healthy and unlikely to get sick from this infection, but if your community, city and country are on lockdown, you will suffer socially and economically. If our health care systems are overloaded, you may not get care when you need it, even for other ailments. Moreover, you may infect your grandparents or a friend battling cancer, causing them harm or even death.

Countries that fail to contain spread may face isolation from the rest of the world, with their borders closed from the outside. Concealing cases now to maintain social normalcy may not be the best option. A tourist destination island may well get one more shipload of tourists through the downtown-shopping district, only to spend millions of dollars later treating their infected population.

Accurate and informative knowledge of this disease, including some of the complicated parts, will help individuals and leaders make better-informed decisions. The next chapters are going to acquaint, or re-acquaint, you with the fundamentals of cell and viral biology to build a common understanding of how humans and viruses affect each other in this ancient battle.

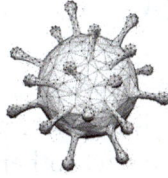

ALL THE MOVING PARTS

The building blocks of biology are carbon-based structures. This is the subject matter of Biochemistry. Fats are used to create membranes that encircle the whole cell, as well as creating smaller internal closed spaces (organelles) within the cell, where specialized work can be done. Sugars and proteins are the other main biochemical structures used in life. While all three of them are incorporated into cell structures, they can also be metabolized to release energy.

Proteins form the movable parts in cells. A protein is a sequence of amino acids joined together. The sequence is carefully folded to make a specific shape. It is the protein shape, and how it can be changed, which forms the movement and very *livingness* of life. Seen from this perspective, running is just a complex set of protein shape changes.

All living creatures are defined by the protein recipes they inherit and the proteins they make from those recipes. There are 22 different amino acids in nature. Humans use 21. Mathematically, the number of different amino acid sequence combinations is literally endless. Each new sequence makes a different protein. The sequence instructions are kept in DNA codes – the very recipe of life.

The Basics of Genetics

DNA codes are built with nucleic acids. Nucleic acids are the fourth major biochemical group essential for Life. There are four different nucleic acids, two in each group of attracted-to-each-other base pairs. Nucleic acids, held together by a sugar/phosphate backbone, can be joined in any sequence and any length of sequence. Each sequence of three nucleic acids in a row, called a codon, forms a code for an amino acid. When there are four different nucleic acids available (4^3), 64 different codons (sequences of three) are possible.

With 64 different codon sequences and only 21 amino acids to code for, all of the amino acids have more than one codon code. For example, the amino acid leucine has six different codons. Three of the codons code for 'stop', or end of protein sequence, and one codes for 'start'. While computer code is binary, *life code* uses *four* bases, with a sequence of three bases (codon) coding for each of the 21 amino acids.

In order to stabilize and protect the code, another set of nucleic acids pair up opposite their respective base pair partners, essentially forming an opposite anti-parallel sequence that closes off the codons and prevents them from interacting with other substances. We call these positive and negative strands that are joined together to create the famous double-stranded DNA, which is then twisted into a helix shape and coated with protective proteins. The opposite code serves to seal the sequence from outside harm, as disruption would alter the code. The codons in our chromosomes encode the amino acid sequences that make up the thousands of different proteins in our bodies.

Our DNA is the set of master-copies of codes for all the proteins we are able to build. We only use 2% of our DNA library to code for all the proteins in our bodies. The rest of the DNA is either 'junk' DNA that we think is no longer used, or form control systems that enable gene sequences to be located, opened and copied (transcribed).

The Basics of Epigenetics

In nucleated cells like ours, our chromosomes are protected inside a nuclear membrane envelope. When a cell senses the need for a particular protein it sends a messenger to bind to receptors on the nuclear membrane. Nuclear receptors, in turn, instruct the nucleus to open and run off a copy of the DNA sequence that will be used to assemble the protein. In this way, the cell controls which proteins are made by only ordering the DNA copies it needs. The nucleus and its DNA do have some say regarding *if*, and *how easily*, they provide copies.

Thus, cells are instructed by their environment and each other to perform according to a whole-body master plan. Stem cells literally wait for instructions to specialize and start working. Working cells get feedback on the needs of the whole organism, combining those signals with their own internal needs, to satisfy both requirements. Old and tired cells signal their distress and, if they cannot make repairs, they may die gracefully (apoptosis) or tragically (necrosis). Occasionally, a cell may develop a perplexing response and become a cancer cell.

To be successful, all creatures must replicate themselves. They must have offspring or they will become extinct. Bacteria come from a long unbroken line of cloning, reaching back to when life began. We too, replicate ourselves by creating a new single cell organism with its treasured DNA copies enclosed. The critical difference, though, is that we, unlike bacteria, are a composite mix of genes from both of our parents. Combining shared DNA from two parents enables gene selection and better long-term survival.

The cell instructs the nucleus when its gene codes are required. When the signal is accepted, the target gene is opened and replicated, making an exact copy of the sequence in an exportable form known as RNA. Each RNA sequence is a copy of the DNA recipe for one particular protein. Assembling proteins requires oxidative chemical reactions between each amino acid in the sequence. Oxidative reactions are harmful to surrounding structures, so RNA is transferred out to the cell for processing, away from the delicate DNA master copies inside the nucleus.

Gene Transcription

RNA is run through an exquisite protein assembly machine called a ribosome. Ribosomes read RNA sequences at incredible speed and with superb accuracy, matching up amino acids according to the code. The amino acids are joined together in sequence by oxidation reactions. The assembled proteins are then transferred to another site in the cell, the endoplasmic reticulum, where they are folded in an exact sequence of folds and clipped into place by further carefully choreographed oxidative reactions. Minerals such as magnesium and zinc may be added as required. Finally, the newly shaped protein is checked for faults and transported to where it is needed, hopefully right on schedule.

Reliability of this transcription system entails keeping control over the ribosomes, making sure that *only* nuclear mandated RNAs are processed. When foreign RNA scripts enter the cell, such as viral RNA, the ribosome can be induced to make foreign proteins that are not derived from its own cell's DNA code.

At the very beginning of life, before even proteins and their DNA recipes had evolved, RNA was the basis of coding and signaling. These RNA sequences are still shared between cells. They can switch off DNA transcription in the nucleus or degrade nuclear RNA transcripts before they reach the ribosome, essentially cancelling transcript orders. We can't survive without this system and we are just beginning to understand it.

Although there is a steady hum of RNA chatter going on in every cell, things get stirred up when an imposter RNA sequence enters the cell and takes over the ribosome equipment. By supplanting a cell's RNA sequence, the imposter RNA is able to make its own proteins, without engaging the hard work of being a living cell.

A successful imposter RNA sequence copy must be able to escape with its newfound cloned family and have at least one of them reach another host cell. From there it's a matter of 'rinse and repeat' for an eternity. The challenge for the imposter RNA is to adjust its strategy just enough to stay ahead of the host cell's attempts to drive it off.

The adage 'if something can be done, it probably has been' is as true of nature as it is in life. The insidious RNA imposters are *viruses* and they are found in all species, including bacteria.

We are at a critical point in our story. The stage is set to delve into the parts of our physiology that are affected by CoV2. Since our aim is to learn about COVID-19, both the host and the virus need to be understood, together and apart, to make sense of this pandemic. Bear with me as we review the part of our physiology that Cov2 has targeted with such devastating effects.

The Evolution of Complex Life

Evolution made a giant leap from simple bacteria and their pesky viruses when two distinct types of cells teamed up and formed a partnership, allowing one cell to live within the other. This unicellular partnership evolved for almost a billion years until it was efficient and stable enough to form multi-cellular organisms. When co-operatives of cells work together for a common good, individual cells are able to specialize, allowing them to take on specific roles. Along with differentiation comes the need for communication. Although each cell must still see to its own internal needs, it must also contribute to the welfare of the whole organism. Co-operation requires information to be shared throughout the organism on a continuous basis.

Over the past few years, I have been trying to understand the different systems in our body and how they work individually and collectively to shape our bodies in response to stress. I sought to pinpoint the fundamental natural stresses that all living cells have endured since the beginning of life and how they sense and respond to those stresses.

One of these fundamental systems is tasked with maintaining the external seawater-like environment that bathes all living cells. It is a vital sensing, communication and response system that engages different organs to maintain the critical composition of interstitial fluid. The majority of us suffer from varying degrees of stress on this system and it is not surprising that its adverse effects contribute to most of our modern diseases. What is surprising is that we are only just beginning to understand this system in some depth.

The 2003 CoV1 mutation took advantage of this system and further CoV2 improvements are the basis for the great harm that Covid-19 is causing us.

Renin Angiotensin System (RAS)

The renin-angiotensin system (RAS) forms an ancient communication system, preserved throughout evolution that regulates a wide range of critical functions including blood flow, salt and water levels and inflammation. It literally ensures that each cell in every organ is provided with enough oxygen and salted interstitial fluid. Cells evolved in seawater which has relatively stable levels of salts and oxygen and all complex organisms must still maintain the same optimal seawater environment that their cell biology evolved in.[3]

The RAS enables every cell in the body to *signal* when they are in distress from sub-optimal oxygen and interstitial fluid levels, which evokes powerful and rapid homeostatic responses to correct those deficiencies. As a result, individual cells are able to demand an increase in blood flow when required.

Although localized blood flow changes can be made by dilating or constricting blood vessels in tissue, systemic-wide changes require the heart, lungs and kidneys to respond to the overall demands from the body. Both the blood vessel dilating endothelial control system and the RAS work in concert.

The RAS stress signal protein that can be made in any cell that is stressed is called angiotensinogen (AGT). Since most AGT is produced in response to low blood flow through the liver, the liver acts as a sensor and regulator of blood flow throughout the body. When another part of the body has inadequate blood flow, it too can message for increased flow. The brain, being as important as it is, has its own control system that is separate from, and overrides, the RAS when it requires higher blood pressure.

In people who are overweight, large fat cells in over-abundant fat (adipose) tissue are very poorly oxygenated. Large fat cells hardly get enough oxygen through their relatively small surface areas and this is compounded by poor blood flow through the scanty blood vessels found in adipose. As a result fat cells produce AGT, lots of it. Adipose can double or triple the total body AGT signal, causing high systemic blood pressure and salt and water retention in an attempt to increase blood flow.[4]

This is why the best way to lower blood pressure is still to exercise and lose weight. Both of those activities lower fat-derived AGT and decreases salt and fluid retention and the resulting hypertension.

AGT is a large protein that must be activated (cleaved) by renin, a protease protein that is made in the kidney. The need for AGT cleavage by renin enables the kidney to have input into the RAS system. A kidney that has poor blood flow, or is vitamin D deficient, increases production of renin, while an unstressed kidney lowers renin production, which reduces the effective AGT stress signal.

Renin cleaves the 485 amino acid AGT down to a 10-amino acid peptide called angiotensin I (AngI). AGT that is oxidized is more easily cleaved by renin, which explains why anti-oxidants themselves lower the RAS stress signal and provides us with, yet, another reason to eat well. The remaining 475-amino acid protein is called des(AngI)AGT and we still don't know if it does anything. Perhaps when we find out we will give it a better name.

AngI is an inactive intermediary protein that must be cleaved again. The second cleavage is done by different proteases throughout the body. This enables different proteases to each produce different proteins from AngI, creating a complex system of variable signals. Every medical student knows that angiotensin-converting enzyme (ACE) cleaves AngI to form angiotensin II (AngII), the final messenger of distress that then binds to AngII receptors.

We used to think that conversion of AngI to AngII was irreversible and that once AngI was formed it exerted uncontrolled downstream effects throughout the body. Drugs were developed to block the protease effect of ACE and prevent the conversion of AngI to AngII. So-called 'ACE inhibitors' are still widely used to treat high blood pressure today by reducing the powerful RAS stress signal.

There is a major flaw in this simplistic treatment approach. Lowering blood pressure just deprives the poorly perfused adipose tissue that initiated the AngII signal in the first place of adequate blood flow, further increasing their AGT stress signals. Biology is rarely linear.

Poorly perfused tissue is under extreme stress and stressed cells do not suffer in silence. They evoke system-wide alarm systems that get stronger as their stress increases or is not alleviated. Hypoxic adipose tissue first increases expression of AGT and then activates inflammatory signals, as the cells literally cry out for help. Hypoxic cells critically need more blood flow to replenish oxygen and interstitial fluid, or they will die. In fact, many fat cells within large adipose deposits do die every day, with the dead cells initiating inflammatory cascades of their own.

Cells and tissues that respond to the AGT stress signal express the AngII receptors AT1 & AT2. Different AT-expressing cells respond in their own way to AT activation but create a coordinated response that increases salt and water retention, blood flow and interstitial fluid levels throughout the body.

This is how obesity causes stress, as it uses the powerful RAS to drive the heart and lungs to work to sustain oxygenation of the excess adipose tissue. We have to work really hard to keep those extra pounds alive. Fat cells also switch on inflammation to increase blood vessel growth in their tissues and to dispose of dead and decaying fat cells.

Fat cells do make an effort not to enlarge too much by becoming resistant to the demands of insulin to take up and store more glucose and fat. They are literally full to bursting, already. This is when the patient is said to develop diabetes, with a high blood sugar level despite having enough insulin in the blood. We call this insulin-resistant type two diabetes.

Humans with excessive RAS activity exhibit the classic phenotype disease called metabolic syndrome, which is characterized by obesity, hypertension, cardiovascular disease and diabetes.

Excessive RAS induces disease in its target cardiovascular, pulmonary and renal systems. Chronic high blood pressure is the first change that reflects increased RAS activity. Chronic high blood pressure causes the blood vessels to remodel the constricting muscles in their walls, while the slippery endothelial cells become inflamed and start to trap white blood cells. Although the heart initially enlarges to increase its pumping performance, it subsequently loses its ability to contract effectively, resulting in heart failure.

The kidneys, too, show signs of injury, with thickening of their filters (glomerulosclerosis) and leakage of proteins. This is referred to as nephropathy. Diabetics commonly experience these changes and frequently go on to suffer complete renal failure and require dialysis treatments.

In the lungs, RAS stress causes enhanced vascular permeability, increased lung water, white blood cell accumulation and worsening of lung function. This is commonly referred to as chronic obstructive lung disease (COPD) and is a precursor to respiratory failure.[5]

The picture that is emerging is one of obesity and lack of exercise, both individually and together, activating RAS stress and the resulting spectrum of metabolic diseases. This brings us to the realization that RAS stress can only be properly addressed at its source and humans are going to have to exercise regularly and lose weight if they hope to be healthy.

The RAS is a sensing system that causes the body to adapt in connected ways in order to survive the extreme stress of being obese and living a sedentary lifestyle. We also force this deranged lifestyle on the animals we raise to eat in order that they might gain as much weight as quickly as possible.

The changes that occur in response to this stress are phenotypic in nature, as we force our bodies to behave in ways that result in bodies that were never intended for life on earth.

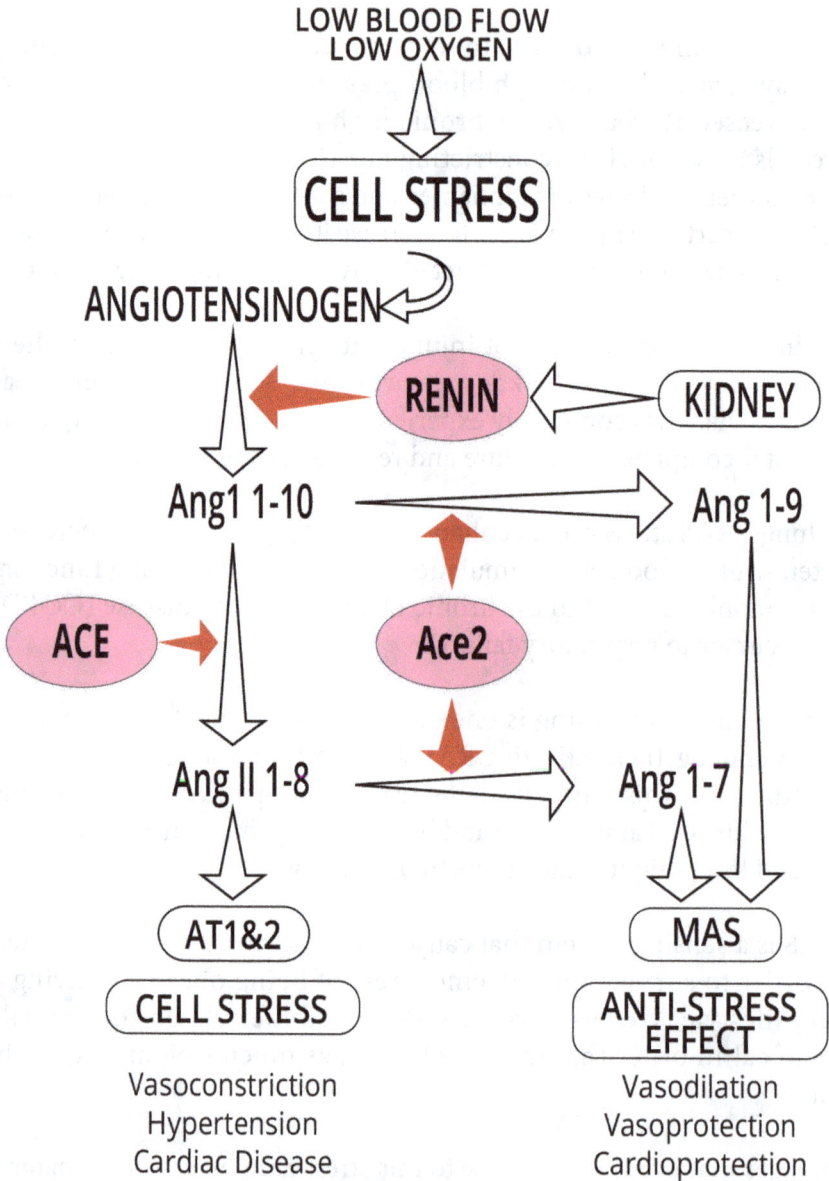

CELL STRESS

LOW BLOOD FLOW
LOW OXYGEN

⬇

CELL STRESS

ANGIOTENSINOGEN

RENIN ⬅ KIDNEY

Ang1 1-10 ➡ Ang 1-9

ACE ➡

Ace2

Ang II 1-8 ➡ Ang 1-7

AT1&2

MAS

CELL STRESS

ANTI-STRESS EFFECT

Vasoconstriction
Hypertension
Cardiac Disease

Vasodilation
Vasoprotection
Cardioprotection

Scientists only recently discovered that the RAS has a built-in rescue system that can tone down many of the stress effects in our heart and lungs. They discovered it just a few years before CoV1 took advantage of it too.

How Ace2 Down-Regulates RAS Stress

Researchers discovered another angiotensin converting enzyme 2 (Ace2) in the late 1990s. Ace2 is also a protease and, like ACE, also cleaves AngI and AngII, except it converts them into the *anti-inflammatory counterparts* Ag1-9 and Ag1-7 respectively. These Ace2-cleaved proteins target a completely different cell receptor (Mas) that has anti-stress effects.[5]

Protease activity of Ace2 provides a critical diversion pathway to modify the RAS stress signal, a signal that we previously thought was irreversible. RAS editing by Ace2 does not prevent the heart from reacting but it prevents a harmful over-reaction. The heart is still driven to work harder, but not hard enough to cause catastrophic failure. In this way, Ace2 slows down the rate of progression of heart disease.[6]

It should come as no surprise then, that Ace2 has been found to play a harm-reduction role in patients with metabolic syndrome. It is important to grasp that the increased Ace2 levels in patients with metabolic syndrome are not contributing to the disease, but are there to reduce it.[7,8]

The RAS stress signal is best used for temporary adjustments to body function, such as tiding things over until we get up in the morning and go for a walk to find water. RAS stress is switched off as soon blood flow is increased enough to satisfy tissue fluid and oxygen requirements and is easily achieved with regular exercise and by staying slim. In its evolutionary role, Ace2 could have helped during prolonged immobilization such as hibernating in winter or temporary obesity such as overeating before winter, where the stress signal persisted for longer periods of time.

Many of us now voluntarily suffer the same life-long immobilization and obesity that our domestic farm animals do. This taxes the RAS to maintain perfusion of continually resting muscles and densely packed adipose tissue.

Instead of dealing with the problem by losing weight and exercising, we increasingly resort to pharmacological solutions in a vain attempt to blunt the effects of RAS stress, without lowering AGT production at the source. Even though our medications merely modify the measurable markers of RAS stress such has high blood sugar, high blood pressure, high cholesterol and increased inflammation, we wonder why the *effects* of metabolic syndrome continue unabated.

Immobility and obesity increases RAS signaling. When this becomes chronic, the cells that are programmed to respond to the AngII signal resort to making Ace2 proteases to reduce their stress to a more tolerable level. Increased Ace2 expression is a local defense mechanism against a systemic RAS stress signal.

RAS stress is just one of six phenotypic maladaptations that harm our health. By not understanding this stress system we have created a faulty narrative and equally faulty methods to restore it. How could we have got it right when we discovered ACE over 50 years ago but not the other half of the story, Ace2, until only 20 years ago?

People living with chronic RAS stress rely increasingly and unknowingly on their Ace2 proteins to keep this stress in check. Unfortunately, when CoV2 uses Ace2 to gain entry to our cells it destroys the vital protease in the process.

COVID-19 is essentially an *acute Ace2 deficiency syndrome* brought on by a zoonotic cold virus that has been gifted to us by bats for the third time this century. Humans relying heavily on the actions of Ace2 to reduce their metabolic stress are at greater risk of severe illness and death, when their Ace2 function is disrupted by a CoV2 infection.

⚜

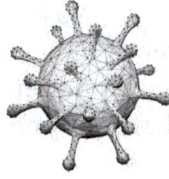

THE ENEMY

T his chapter will review how viruses and coronaviruses, in particular, go about their business. The first section will cover the basics of microbes and viruses before reviewing coronaviruses in general and each of the three new coronaviruses that have emerged this century.

What is a virus?

A virus is one of the most basic forms of biological matter and is the very epitome of a parasite. It reproduces itself by invading a living cell and hijacking that cell's biology for its own ends. First, a virus must find a way to enter a cell. Next, it must evade detection and destruction long enough to induce the cell to make its viral proteins and RNA in order to assemble them into exact copies of itself, complete with a method of escape. Viral replication is an intricate and parasitic way of cloning.

In order to be successful, a virus must adapt to the lifecycle of its host species. It must survive the trip between hosts and put itself in contention to be picked up by the next host. This lifecycle may not rely on hurting or killing the host. On the contrary, there is seldom any benefit from killing its host as viral replication relies on healthy living cells, not dead biological matter.

A virus is not a bacterium, those tiny living cells we call microbes. Bacteria are very small single-cell organisms that are alive. Bacteria have a cell membrane inside a cell wall that creates a barrier against the outside world with a carefully controlled layer of interstitial fluid between them. They absorb nutrients and excrete waste and reproduce themselves by dividing into two equal parts once they have become large enough.

Bacteria that divide rapidly can outnumber their competitors and in so doing, have a better chance of survival. However, they must replicate their whole DNA code before they can divide, so the less DNA they have the quicker they can divide. In order to win the race to divide, bacteria continually strip down their DNA to the bare necessities.

Stripping down DNA reduces DNA diversity. Although their genes do mutate randomly, bacteria don't rely on mutations as a strategy for survival. Instead bacteria share their genes with other bacteria in a process called *lateral gene transfer*. Gene sharing enables bacteria to adapt to diverse environments and pass on that capability to other bacteria.

A bacterium is not a virus. A virus is simply a collection of genetic code wrapped up in a protein envelope. The viral envelope protects genetic code when the virus is outside its host cell and enables the virus to enter a prospective host cell. A virus has a small genome that codes for the few proteins needed in its brief lifecycle. This lifecycle entails entering its host cell and using that cell's apparatus to copy its proteins and RNA codes, which are then assembled into replicated 'selves'. A virus also keeps its own genome small by using as many host cell proteins and systems as possible.

The Life Cycle of a Virus

Viruses have been around since the beginning of life. They have evolved to ensure their survival by continual replication in host cells, without ever developing the means to function autonomously. They are the quintessential parasite and so deeply enmeshed in nature that we can't exist without them.

The parasitic lives of viruses have not gone unnoticed by their hosts. In fact, cells put a great deal of effort into defending themselves against viruses.

A defenseless cell could be commandeered by a virus to produce its proteins to exhaustion.

All living cells know how to kill viruses. Plants even know how to kill viruses. No organism can be alive in 2020 without an inherent ability to kill invading viruses! We are just beginning to understand the complex game of cat-and-mouse that viruses and their hosts play.

Viral Spread

Viruses spread and infect new hosts continuously. Spreading is the very essence of success for a virus, not its ability to find food. We've already seen that this is not the same for bacteria, which rely on rapid replication to stay ahead of the competition.

To spread, a virus must find another living creature and *use that animal's cells to clone itself* before moving on. Put scientifically, a virus must replicate in the primary host, be excreted from the host in some intermediary material and be transmitted to a secondary host. Every virus on earth today has survived an unbroken chain of infecting and cloning stretching back billions of years.

Cloning itself takes time. We call this the incubation period. It is the interval between admission to the first cell and detection by the infected host. That's the point when 'all hell breaks loose'. The incubation period gives the unwitting host time to move from the site where the virus was encountered. The longer the incubation period and the faster and farther the hosts move, the wider the virus spreads. The popularity of air travel has helped us become viral super-spreaders.

During a long trans-continental flight a newly infected passenger may enter the transmission phase of their viral illness and start spewing millions of new viruses during the flight. Sometime later, the host cells might sound the alarm and cause the traveller to feel sick. At this point, our weary traveller might still not recognize these symptoms to be the first signs of illness. After all, who does feel great on a fourteen-hour flight? They can be forgiven for not heeding those early warnings and dismissively thinking; "Let me just get to my hotel room, have a hot shower and take a nap."

Meanwhile, the virus spreads in the crowded plane by way of re-circulating airflow. Hours later dozens of newly infected hosts disembark onto a different continent, some headed to urban destinations while other travellers wait in the airport departure lounge for connecting flights to exotic and unsuspecting remote places. Viruses have become beneficiaries of human ingenuity that makes the scope and speed of their spread almost unfathomable.

It is a useful strategy for viruses to begin spreading before the host feels sick. Some viruses have completed many rounds of replication and have viral shedding well underway before the host cells are alerted and mount a response. In this situation, the prodromal period (no symptoms) and the infectious stage (spreading) overlap. When a virus begins spreading *before* symptoms appear in the host, it can be highly contagious.

Viral spread around the host body is easy to imagine. Newly hatched viruses circulate in blood or spread locally from cell to cell. Transition to a new host can be precarious and most viruses die during the crossing. Their survival depends on the toughness of their envelope but ultimately requires a secondary host to ingest or inhale excretions of the primary host.

Measuring Spread

The rate of viral spread and whether the spread becomes self-sustaining is represented scientifically by a measured ratio called the *basic reproduction number (R-0)*. You will hear it spoken as "R–naught" or "R-zero". R-0 is defined as the average number of secondary cases generated in a susceptible population. For a virus to keep spreading, the primary host must infect more than one other person. In other words, the R-0 must be above 1. The better the virus is able to spread, the higher its R-0 is. An R-0 over 2 is moderate spread, above 3 is highly contagious and above 4 is scary.

In this basic reproduction R-0 setting, where primary and secondary hosts are unaware of the presence of the virus, neither are making a conscious effort *to avoid* transmitting the virus. They are all just going about their normal business. The susceptible population can be passengers in an airplane or represent all the humans in a city or country. We've seen that being cooped up in a plane or on a cruise ship is losing its allure.

The R-0 reflects the *potential* for spread before control measures are in place, reflecting what would happen if we *did nothing* and just let nature run its course. Basic reproduction happens in unsuspecting communities. Today, much of Africa is in the R-0 phase as there are people there who have not been told that Cov2 has arrived, no cases have been identified and no contagion prevention measures are in place.

The R-0 of the virus reduces sharply once the infection declares itself and the hosts change their behavior to reduce infection. Defensive actions by the population changes R-0 to the *effective reproduction number (R-t)*.

R-t can be lowered in a number of ways. Firstly, the number of susceptible people is reduced when some of them become infected and either die or recover and develop immunity. Secondly, effective control measures can be implemented to contain the spread. In order to contain the epidemic, the R-t must be reduced as much as possible, preferably without much contribution from dying.

To end an outbreak the R-t must be brought below 1, indicating that the infected population is infecting fewer new people. At this time of writing in early 2020, humanity is collectively catching its breath as each new day shows the COVID-19 numbers rising around the world. We all hope for the numbers to peak, indicating that the rate of spread is dropping below the crucial R-t of 1.

Although the R-t was quickly brought below 1 with SARS, we may not be so lucky this time. There are two things working against us. First, SARS patients only started spreading their viruses after they started feeling sick and developed a fever, providing an immediate warning to quarantine.

Second, *everyone* who was infected with the SARS virus got sick. There were no silent spreaders.

This time is different. First, it appears that there is a significant lag-time between becoming infectious and developing symptoms. Under these circumstances, spread will stay high and not be controlled using only the reactionary measures used during SARS. Second, some of us may not get much in the way of symptoms at all. While they may be considered the fortunate ones, they unknowingly host and spread the virus with minimal illness. In this setting, the virus can revert to its innate spreading ability, which is proving to be quite impressive.

Entry into Host Cells

Entry into the target cell is the first critical step for a virus to infect a new host. A virus cannot simply push its way into a cell, as cell membranes are impermeable to viruses; however, cell membranes are studded with thousands of different proteins that are put there (expressed) by the cell to communicate and interact with their surroundings. About a third of the proteins that are encoded in our DNA are destined to be membrane proteins.

A membrane protein's function depends on its shape and its ability to interact with other molecules and change its shape. Let's take the calcium pumping protein as an example. Our cells pump calcium continuously throughout our lives. A membrane protein that pumps calcium first binds to a calcium ion which enables it to accept an energized phosphate ion from adenosine triphosphate (ATP), the roving cellular 'rechargeable batteries'. Phosphate binding (phosphorylation) changes the protein's shape, causing it to involute itself and deposit the calcium ion on the *other side* of the membrane.

There are thousands of proteins expressed on every cell's membrane. Each cell expresses the proteins that are needed to make that cell perform its intended function. A virus's outer lipoprotein envelope must be able to interact with one of those membrane proteins if it is to successfully access a host cell. Although many of these proteins are common to a variety of species, their exact shape may differ enough that the virus cannot interact with them. This is why viruses cannot simply jump to another species. Equally, only minor changes in the viral envelope proteins may change its ability to enter a cell. The SARS and MERS viruses changed relatively few gene sequences in their envelope protein codes to become grave threats to humans.

Even viruses that are closely related and have almost identical genes, may differ just enough to prevent zoonotic cross-infection. Equally, they may cross over into other species with similar receptors by changing their envelope proteins just enough to make the leap.

The successful virus must bind to a host receptor and be transported into the cell. Once inside the cell, the viral RNA or DNA separates from the transport protein, the cell membrane and its own envelope to start cloning itself.

Replication

Once inside and undressed, the replicating cycle begins. Some things never change! The virus must first take over the protein assembly machinery of the cell to makes proteins that form an ad-hoc replicating complex to make copies of the viral gene sequences.

It is during this hectic replication process that the gene sequences can be miscopied (mutated) to create subtly different viruses. Small coding errors occur when the reverse image nucleotide partner is mismatched, creating a one-nucleotide mistake in a 4-nucleotide codon. When this happens, a different amino acid may replace the original one and change the protein structure and its function.[9]

Newly formed viral proteins are assembled into a virus, essentially a clone that is then coated in an envelope and escorted to the cell membrane for release.

Despite a cell's best efforts to hamper viral activities, their detection avoidance strategies make the coronavirus a formidable foe. Detailing these strategic mechanisms is beyond the scope of this book. Suffice to say, their techniques are complex and intricate and are still being worked out in order for us to develop ways of thwarting viral proliferation.

☙

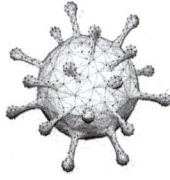

HOW WE RESPOND

Innate Cell Defense

Host cell defense strategies depend of detecting viral proteins that the virus uses to replicate itself. The protein machinery set up by the virus to run the 'grow-op' is readily recognized as foreign. The virus, in turn, employs elaborate techniques to disguise its 'grow-op' proteins and conceal them from the innate immune sensors. Again, some things never change![9]

A virus must replicate its RNA during cloning in a process that requires the formation of double-stranded RNA, something host cells never do. Reliably recognizing double-stranded viral RNA is part of their defense strategy.

As viral RNA codes are run through host ribosomes, transcribed proteins are transported to the endoplasmic reticulum (ER) for folding. Heavy protein-folding demand stresses the cell and activates an innate stress response. The virus tries to slow down the protein folding process and avoid detection of its nefarious activities.

Cellular self-destruction is the primary method of defense in the face of an overwhelming virus infection in order to prevent runaway viral replication. If cells are already stressed before a viral infection, then they may overreact and self-destruct when only mildly infected. Since older hosts innately have more ER stress, this may explain why viral infections are not well tolerated by the elderly.

Innate cell defense uses an array of intra-cellular sensor proteins. Sensor activation results in gene transcription to make defensive proteins, which include inflammatory cytokines and viral-killing interferon. Interferon proteins target virtually every step of the viral cycle and restrict viral replication.

Innate cellular immunity detects and destroys viruses within the cell as well as activating the adaptive immune system to mount a whole-body response to clear viruses outside the cell. Much of the illness associated with viral infections is brought on by the immune response.

This really is inter-protein warfare - but our cells *do* have a winning strategy. We know that plants have learned to counter viruses and they, too, make substances that interrupt the lifecycles of viruses. It should come as no surprise that we may find help in the garden in our fight against Cov2.

Fever

During the incubation phase of a viral infection, the cell response has been a domestic dispute played out behind the closed doors of the cell membrane. When the cells' collective defensive efforts cannot contain the spread of infection, they produce cytokines that call for back-up from the real heroes at times like these, the white blood cells, and the whole body responds in a concerted way.

Initially, the brain raises our body temperature and we get a **fever**. That is why a raised temperature is usually first sign of an infection. At about the same time, we develop a fever, viruses begin leaving our cells in droves and can be detected in our body fluids by a viral detection kit that can identifies the virus by its RNA signature.

Fever is the hallmark of an activated immune system, whatever the cause. It is a defensive response designed to promote the activity of our immune cells, while hampering the cloning activities of the invaders. Most animals respond to infection with a fever.

Cytokines signal the temperature setting center in the hypothalamus of the brain by attaching to receptors in the blood vessels in the brain and causing them to make another set of inflammatory molecules called *prostaglandins*. Prostaglandins relay the inflammatory signals into the deep brain structures, raising the temperature set point and causing the body to warm itself up to the higher temperature. That is why we shiver and cover ourselves up.[10]

The cytokine surge and the fever it causes are a general *call-to-arms*. The fight is on. Time to get into bed and let the battle rage.

Immune System Response

Once the immune system is activated, cascades of powerful protein signals are unleashed. Inflammatory responses can be powerful enough to kill us, as evidenced by an anaphylactic reaction to something as innocuous as a peanut.

The immune system response relies on white blood cells being activated. Circulating monocytes heed the call and migrate into the infected part of the body where they transform themselves into macrophage cells that can engulf infected and dying cells. While digesting the infected cells, they pick out the viral proteins from the debris and express them on their cell membranes. Although an unseemly image, it's like hanging the dead bodies of a defeated enemy in the market square for everyone to see.

The viral antigens presented on the macrophage's outer surface are detected by lymphocytes, another type of white blood cell. Having avoided the dirty digesting work done by macrophages, lymphocytes absorb the presented antigen and use it to form a template to create an antibody protein that will attach to it.

The lymphocyte then passes on this precious information to two other types of white cells. One is the CD8 killer lymphocyte that targets heavily infected cells for elimination and the other is the B-lymphocyte that produces antibody proteins to immobilize the virus.

When circulating antibodies bind to the antigen protein sequence on a live virus, they harm or destroy the virus. Antibody proteins also act like handcuffs on the virus and encourage macrophages to engulf the antibody-virus complex and destroy it.

When this works well, the infection is cleared without too much harm. In some cases, many infected host cells are destroyed and explains why we need time to recover after an illness. The fight really is a war of attrition.

ABO Blood Group Antibodies

One well-known antibody system relates to our blood group. Red blood cells have distinct proteins attached to their surface that can be recognized as foreign proteins when the blood is transfused into another person; hence they are called *antigens.* There are two possible antigens in the ABO blood group system, A and B. Their presence determines an individual's blood group designation as either A, B, AB (when both antigens are present), or O when neither is present.

Having the antigens on our red cells blocks our immune system from making antibodies to them. Group O patients who have neither antigen develop antibodies to both the A and B antigens. Conversely, AB patients do not have either antibody. Group A patients have anti-B antibodies and group B patients have anti-A antibodies.

It turns out that these antibodies are useful for a number of health reasons, including fighting off coronaviruses. During the SARS epidemic and now during Covid-19, researchers identified a significantly better outcome in patients who were group O, and worse outcome in group A patients. These clinical outcomes support the laboratory finding that anti-A antibodies do specifically inhibit the adhesion of SARS-CoV viruses to the target Ace2 enzyme in humans.[11]

People with group-O blood are expected to fare better from Covid-19 than those with group-A blood type.

Vaccines

A vaccine is essentially a pseudo-infection. It is usually a mild or weakened form of the disease-causing virus that is safe to inject as it is easily overcome by our immune system. The attenuated version of the virus must contain the same target protein-sequence as the virus being vaccinated against. Our immune cells find a signature protein sequence of the virus and our B-lymphocytes make antibodies to that sequence.

Antibodies target the outside of viruses; therefore the target protein sequence needs to be part of the viral envelope. Vaccine scientists tear viruses apart and try to figure which piece will make a good antigen target. They use a combination of science and artful trial-and-error to induce antibody production in us. Memory cells also need to be induced to *remember the antibody code* so that they can activate antibody production as soon as the real infection starts.

If a patient is *already* infected, then it is too late to induce an antibody response with a vaccine, especially if the virus attacks fast. Fortunately, rabies is a slow onset viral disease that can be treated with a vaccine if it is given soon after the bite of a rabid animal.

Serum

Antibodies made by other live animals or cell cultures grown in a laboratory can help us fight off an infection, but humans who have already survived the infection and have high antibody levels to it are the best source of antibodies. The antibodies are separated from whole blood to remove unwanted red blood cells. This separated fraction of blood, which is called serum or plasma, can then be safely injected into a newly infected patient.

During this epidemic we may see more reliance on antibody serum from survivors than ever before. Those of us who survive will have an opportunity help others by donating blood so that precious antibody-laden serum can be extracted and used.

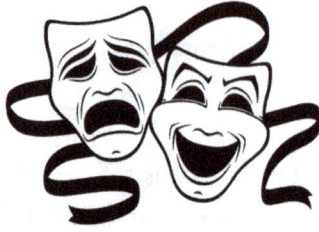

SAMSARA

*"And, like this insubstantial pageant faded" ***

we are nothing but costumed players
this performance that scene; all judged and all graded
artifice and acting down all the human layers
still what joy it is to wear this jaunty mask
and to play to pitch perfection this famous role
surely it is in the ways and weight of the world not too much to ask
that this players game should not be so burdensome on the soul
for if the role is played well, do you think anyone cares who you really are?
and that by peeling back the façade you will be able to escape this players game?
maybe there is some equanimity found in knowing if you are a footling or a star
so strut forth, on the boards and stage and call out your scripted, imagined made up name
ah a warning. As they say in my current age, you should fake it till you make it
but remember there is always more enterprise in the costume you put on by stripping naked

included with permission from the author: Toby Shannan

* from The Tempest by William Shakespeare

This sonnet, written by a personal friend, is placed here as it deals with
costumes and masks and who we really are underneath it all.
The corona virus is one such masked 'player'.

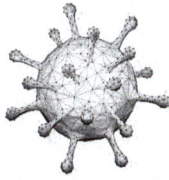

CORONAVIRUS

Overview

Coronaviruses are part of a large family of viruses called Nidovirales that all have an envelope surrounding their positive sense (+) RNA gene codes. They have large RNA *genomes* for a virus, carrying genetic code to make proteins that are used during the replication cycle in host cells.[12]

The coronavirus is spherical with club-shaped spike projections on its envelope surface. It is this envelope that enables the virus to survive so well outside of its host. The Spike (S) protein forms the infamous corona spikes that are used to attach to and enter host cells, essentially acting as a key to the host cell.

Although we have our own endemic coronavirus strains that we have learned to co-exist with, it is quite likely that we have met other zoonotic coronaviruses in the past. I have come to wonder whether our extinct cave-dwelling Neanderthal cousins faced-off against such a zoonotic bat coronavirus, which might have spared us because it couldn't bind to our equivalent entry protein.

Successful viruses often develop long-term relationships with their host species. Our four coronas that plague us were first identified in 1960 and have likely been with us for eons. They are thought to cause about 15-30% of all common colds and are usually only dangerous to newborns, the elderly and the sick. In fact, human coronaviruses were considered to be so harmless that we don't have a vaccine for this old nuisance.

Coronaviruses are found in a wide range of animals besides humans, including many other mammals, fish, birds and snakes and are better known to veterinarians. They cause a range of diseases and target the lungs, gut, liver and brain. There are four main subgroups of coronas: alpha, beta, gamma and delta. The alpha and beta subgroups are only found in mammals where they cause respiratory infections in humans and gut infections in animals.

When a virus crosses into a new animal, the virus may spread a lot better and cause increased disease severity. Bats are a large reservoir of coronaviruses. It seems we first *knowingly* encountered them after a bat-borne coronavirus infected humans in December 2003. Humans have had experiences in the recent past with these viruses, as evidenced by the fact that antibodies to these viruses have been found in people who live near bats.[13]

We have known for over fifty years that coronaviruses *can* and *do* jump species with unpredictable and often disastrous results. When a virus infects a different population, we must ask:

- Did a *mutation* change its entry protein, enabling it to access a species that it was previously in regular but futile contact with?

- Did the virus make a chance crossover to a new species that it was already able to infect, without having to mutate?

A virus that affects a the same population differently poses the question:

- Did the endemic virus *mutate* to alter its virulence?

- Did the host alter its *phenotype* and therefore its ability to cope with the virus?

Remember, the term *phenotype* refers to how we use our genes to react to our environment. While we can't change our genes, we *can* influence which genes we use. To illustrate how this might play out in the face of a viral infection, we might consider whether the Porcine Epidemic Diarrhea Virus that causes severe gastroenteritis in young piglets has the same effect in *wild pigs*, or is it the result of the domestic pigs being caged and overfed?

With all of this in mind, we should consider:

- whether the coronavirus made the leap *unchanged* – simply benefitting from humans getting too close to its natural host habitat.

- whether the coronavirus *mutated* just enough to make the next, not-infrequent, human contact stick.

- whether humans changed their *phenotype* enough to allow the virus to take advantage of their altered lifestyles.

- whether humans tinkered with the virus, creating intentional changes in the RNA sequence by joining up bits of RNA from different viruses.

There is evidence for all four considerations, including the last one. I do not wish to dwell on this any longer, as it is of no consequence now. Virologists and investigators may find answers to some of these questions when this pandemic is over. For now, one thing is clear: we should stay clear of bats.

Since it is obvious that we are changing phenotypically, we need to understand the nature of these changes to determine the implications to both our health and our interactions with old foes like viruses. The concept of altered susceptibility is especially important in light of coronaviruses that are poised to infect us. CoV2 is our third major go-around with a zoonotic coronavirus this century. It is unlikely to be our last.[14]

Up till the end of the 20th century, human coronavirus infections were limited to causing the common cold. Nevertheless, researchers were well aware of the risk posed by pathogenic coronaviruses in animals, particularly bats. The SARS and CoV-like viruses that exist in turtles, pangolins, snakes, civets and raccoon dogs in southern China are thought to have originated in bats.

THE THREE CORONAS

DISEASE	VIRUS	NICKNAME
		(in this book)
SARS	SARS-CoV	CoV1
MERS	MERS-CoV	
COVID-19	SARS-CoV2	CoV2

SARS-CoV (CoV1) and The SARS Epidemic of 2003

SARS-CoV (CoV1), which caused SARS, was the first of the three new coronaviruses to infect humans. It surfaced in November 2002 in Foshan, in the south of China near Hong Kong. Patients began presenting with devastating lung inflammation, a **severe acute respiratory syndrome**, *(SARS)* of unknown cause. The word 'syndrome' means that the cause or mechanism of a disease is unknown.[15]

New cases followed the first Foshan patient, with 300 cases being reported in China by February 2003. One third of those infected were health care workers. As we read in the Prologue of Dr. Ho's first-hand account, the virus spread outside of China when a 64-year-old doctor, who had been directly treating SARS patients, travelled from Guangdong province to a hotel in Hong Kong. It appears that he did not infect anyone en route. The doctor likely only developed symptoms after arriving in Hong Kong, where he infected guests staying on the same floor of his hotel. When the guests went home, they spread the virus to 26 countries in a matter of days.

The high infection rate of SARS became apparent when a single patient who was treated in an open ward for community-acquired pneumonia infected 138 people within 2 weeks of falling ill.

The World Health Organization (WHO) first issued a global alert on March 12, 2003 concerning viral infections in China, Hong Kong and Vietnam. The virus infected 8098 people, killing 774 (10%), all in the space of 6 months.

The initial (R-0) transmission rate of SARS was 2.2 - 3.7 It was highly infectious. What helped mitigate spread was that the virus was transmitted only *after* the patient started to experience symptoms. Viral shedding only occurred during the period the patient felt unwell, making it possible to get the R-t below 1 relatively quickly.

CoV1 was found in sputum, nasal secretions, feces and bronchial washings of infected patients. Transmission occurred by direct contact and coughing and sneezing. Wearing either a surgical or N95-type masks protected health care providers.

Some patients spread their infections more than others. They were termed "super-spreaders". Their heightened infectivity might reflect their lack of infection control precautions and larger amounts of respiratory secretions. Coughing carelessly, when infected, spread the virus more effectively.

Rapid isolation of cases and their contacts enabled SARS to be contained within a few months. The WHO reported on July 5, 2003 that the last know human-to-human transmission of SARS had been broken. Those in the know let out a deep sigh of relief. The rest of the world got on with their business, seemingly oblivious to the threat and barely grateful to all those who had worked and died to contain it. I, too, am shamefully unaware how we honored our Canadian heroes.

Clinical Features of SARS

SARS caused severe pneumonitis or inflammatory infiltration. The virus was later found to have gained access to lung cells by binding to a specific cell receptor found in the respiratory tract, called angiotensin-converting enzyme 2 (Ace2). The two proteins formed a tight bond, causing Ace2 to pull back into the cell, dragging the virus with it.[16]

Interestingly, the Ace2 protein had only recently been discovered a few years earlier and researchers were just coming to grips with it function. Its role in SARS was also only appreciated some time later.

In 2003 the diagnosis of SARS really depended on identifying patient contact with other known cases of SARS. There was no reliable way to positively identify the virus on the spot. Isolating infected patients was the key to containing SARS. Hospitalized patients were subject to strict isolation and barrier nursing to contain spread within the hospital itself.

Symptoms of SARS were quite striking and consistent, including fever (100%), cough (50%) and myalgia (50%). Shortness of breath, headache, diarrhea and nausea and vomiting were less consistent.

The virus targeted the lungs, causing fluid to leak from inflamed blood vessels in the lung. The presence of alveolar fluid made it harder for the lung to absorb oxygen. Maintaining oxygenation was the most important treatment. Attempts to kill the virus likely did not help and might have caused harm.

The patient's immune cytokine response caused fever and muscle ache while lung inflammation and fluid extravasation into the alveoli cause the patient to cough and feel short of breath. The infection was noted for its rapid onset and severity of lung inflammation, which affected 16% of those infected, of which 50% died. Headache and diarrhea/vomiting indicated brain and gut infection respectively.

Treatments for SARS

At the time of the infection, it was not known which treatments might help. Doctors were flying blind. Treatments differed around the world with significant differences in death rates. Canada and Hong Kong had the highest mortality. Since the number of cases was small, it is difficult to draw many conclusions.

A systematic review of all treatments tried during the SARS outbreak includes 366 published studies. Most of these studies were simply descriptions of treatments and outcomes, making it impossible to compare one treatment against a placebo in a matched group of patients; however, older age and the presence of diabetes were consistently found to be associated with a worse outcome.[17]

Corticosteroids

During the SARS outbreak, doctors often turned to steroids in an effort to blunt inflammation and reduce lung fluid. During the critical second week of a SARS infection the patients were at increased risk from lung inflammation while their viral loads were declining rapidly.

Steroid treatment was used *early* in the course of the disease blunted the immune response and aided viral replication, making things worse. When used later, during the pneumonia phase in the critical second week, high dose steroid was associated with a much higher (90%) recovery rate.

Steroids raise blood glucose levels and can cause psychosis. Prolonged high dose steroids caused avascular necrosis of the femoral head (hip) and fungal super-infection was found in the lungs of patients who died. As we read in Dr. Ho's personal account of the SARS outbreak in Hong Kong, high-dose steroid treatment can also cause bowel perforation.

It seems that a short course of high dose steroid withheld until the start of severe respiratory symptoms might have provided the most benefit with the least risk.

Ribavirin (Hepatitis C treatment)

Ribavirin is an intravenous, anti-viral drug that is used to treat hepatitis C and respiratory syncytial virus (RSV) lung infections in children. Although it blocks viral RNA replication, it also blocks host RNA transcription and harms the cell. It is not without side effects.

Despite thirty different reports of ribavirin use, it may not have helped. Ribavirin does cause hemolytic anemia, which lowers patients' hemoglobin levels. Hemoglobin is vital for transporting oxygen and having a low hemoglobin level in the setting of respiratory failure and hypoxia is highly detrimental.

Lopinavar and ritinovar (HIV treatment)

Both drugs are thought to work better when given together and are used in combination to treat HIV infections. Lopinavar has demonstrated benefit in monkey kidney cells infected with coronavirus.

Lopinavar and ritinovar given in combination seemed to help when given early in the course of the infection, especially if combined with ribavirin and steroids; however, the patients chosen to receive treatment may have had a better chance of survival even without the drugs.

Since these two anti-HIV drugs work better in the early phase of the infection and due to the fact that Covid-19 usually presents late in the course of the infection, they will likely not get a call-up for duty in this COVID-19 epidemic.

It will be interesting to see how HIV/Aids patients already on these drugs fare when infected with CoV2.

Interferon

Interferon kills viruses and has been shown to kill CoV1 in a laboratory setting. There are a number of subtypes interferon, and each has a different effect. Overall, it appears that interferon treatment was not very effective in the SARS epidemic, although to be fair, it is difficult to tease out the individual effects of a drug when given with other drugs in small numbers of patients.

IFN-alfacon-1 in combination with high dose steroids showed more rapid lung recovery and may be worth using on patients requiring ventilation, for a short period of time.

Plasma/serum treatment

Using premade viral antibodies is always appealing. Blood plasma from convalescent patients should have sufficient antibody levels to the virus to help patients fighting the infection.

Intravenous immune globulin (IVIG) consists of pooled antibodies from multiple donors, although not from coronavirus survivors. The presumption is that the antibody boost helps modulate and suppress the over-reacting immune system by down-regulating cytokine expression.

Although both IVIG and convalescent plasma were used during SARS, it could not be proven that they were effective. Plasma exchange between a dying patient and a recovered person was done as salvage therapy in Hong Kong, but we can't tell if it worked.

Middle Eastern Respiratory Syndrome (MERS)

MERS-CoV is also a zoonotic virus that resides in bats and is transmitted to humans through camels. Although the virus can be transmitted between humans, new cases usually had close contact with camels themselves. There have been three separate MERS outbreaks and each was easily contained, reflecting a low infection potential. MERS-CoV uses a different host protein to enter a cell; therefore, it causes a different disease response.[18,19]

Although the first case was identified in Jeddah, Saudi Arabia in June 2012, a retrospective analysis of a similar outbreak in April of 2102 in Jordan confirmed that MERS-CoV had in fact caused that outbreak.

The total number of MERS infections totaled 1,593 with 568 deaths. This indicates a death rate of 35%, almost four-fold higher than for SARS. Even though the death rate for MERS was higher than for SARS, the low transmission of the virus and the requirement for animal exposure made this outbreak easier to contain. A third MERS outbreak, in South Korea, was attributed to poor compliance with infection control measures in an abattoir.

Just as with SARS, patients with pre-existing disease had a significantly increased chance of dying. These diseases included obesity, diabetes, chronic cardiac and lung diseases. Immune compromised patients are also at risk.

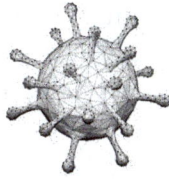

SARS-CoV-2 (CoV2)

Thus far, we have built an understanding of viruses and human responses to infections. The SARS and MERS outbreaks were a prelude to CoV2. Now that coronaviruses are no longer a mystery, we are able to appreciate the remarkable ingenuity of CoV2.

CoV2 is a beta coronavirus in the same family as CoV1. Its closest relatives are CoVZX21 and CoV ZC45, which are both found in bats. The main difference between these viruses is in the genes that code for their surface proteins. This latest change in the surface protein is responsible for the impressive gain-of-function to its spreading ability that increases its virulence.[20]

Spread

In the study of medications (pharmacology), potency refers to how much of a drug is required in order to get an effect. This can depend on how well a drug binds to its target receptor. Potency influences how concentrated a drug needs to be to work. Just as 10mg of morphine is a safe dose of opiate to treat pain, 10mg of the more potent fentanyl will cause death within minutes and the same dose of carfentanyl could kill a whole village.

Potency explains why this viral pandemic has gone from the usual droplet-spread infection that requires close contact with a coughing host, to a possible aerosol infection spread by normal breathing across a room. A droplet is a much larger drop of sputum or saliva that is too heavy to stay aloft in the air for long, whereas smaller aerosol particles can stay aloft for minutes. Equally, a small aerosol particle is much more likely to be inhaled right down into the lung of the next host, instead of being caught in their upper airway and cleared.

Viral envelope proteins serve to protect the virus while in the vulnerable phase between host cells. Having located their target cell after being inhaled, the envelope needs to be opened. Just as a computer virus hiding in an email requires us to open that email before it can infect our computer, this virus also needs to be opened.

Cell Entry

Proteins that cut other proteins are called proteases and are common in all living creatures. We saw how proteases work in the RAS system and we are now going to see how one of those proteases, Ace2, is used by CoV2 to enter those cells expressing Ace2. Many viruses rely on host proteases proteins to cleave their envelopes open to enable cell entry. A virus with a reliable combination of a host protease and a receptor that are easily accessible when it enters its new host will be highly infectious (virulent).

Once opened, the coronavirus must bind to its target receptor. In a similar way that drug affinity affects its potency, the more effectively and reliably a virus binds to its receptor protein, the fewer viruses are needed to establish an infection. This pattern of viral opening before entering has been well established by studying the influenza virus, which uses a very similar technique for gaining entry to our cells, albeit through a different receptor.

Influenza virus mutations often alter their envelope cleavage sites, changing protease action and making the new virus more *or* less potent. This occurred in the 1997 Hong Kong influenza (H5N1) outbreak and a century ago during the Spanish Flu. Ongoing mutations involving their 'break-and-enter' proteins continue to characterize new influenza outbreaks from year to year.[23] Annual outbreaks of new variations of the influenza virus continue to help scientists understand these processes, and how viruses manipulate them.

The CoV2 surface protein is a classic trimeric Spike-protein found in coronaviruses. Trimeric means that is has three separate loosely bonded protein components that are readily cleaved by proteases. When a trimeric protein is pulled apart, the three individual proteins take on a new shape and function differently.

Both CoV1 and 2 are peculiar for their spike protein geometries that are perfectly structured to interact with human Ace2. Unfortunately for us, CoV2 has a 10 – 20 times higher affinity for our Ace2 protein than CoV1, vastly increasing its cell entry capability.[21,22]

There is something else at work here. As CoV2 approaches its target cell, it is literally prepared (primed) for attachment by a second lung protease that is abundant in human lungs. This protease is called **transmembrane protease serine type 2** (TMPRSS2).

As we saw earlier in the RAS system, many cells make protease proteins to cleave other proteins. Proteases are an important part of the complex communication networks in our bodies as they cleave protein messages to activate, divert or alter the message. Proteases also cleave the surface proteins of viruses. In fact, viruses rely on host proteases.

Scientists have been working on the protease system for decades. Protease inhibitor drugs are well known for treating viral infections like HIV, working to inhibit HIV virus envelopes. Chronic pancreatitis and some forms of emphysema also benefit from protease inhibition. The state of our lung proteases determines how susceptible we are to CoV2 infection.

The coronavirus Spike-protein has evolved to have a similar mechanism. Human-infecting coronavirus Spike-proteins are cleaved by proteases at two specific S1/S2 cleavage sites, enabling each segment to re-configure for optimal entry capability.

The S1 protein segment contains an amino acid sequence called the Receptor Binding Domain (RBD) that binds to Ace2. The RBD sequence has only 14 amino acids, of which 6 are common to the RBD of CoV1. *Just 8 amino acid substitutes* are responsible for most of the incredible 'gain-of-function" potency of CoV2.[24]

TMPRSS2 is found with Ace2 in the lung where they both work on the new arrival. TMPRSS2 primes the virus by cleaving the S1 protein at the S1/S2 cleavage site. While the exposed RBD binds to Ace2 the S2 protein with its 2 peptide sequences (fusion and internal fusion peptides) must also be cleaved to enable the virus to cross the cell membrane.[25]

As if in a desperate attempt to fight back against RBD binding, Ace2 (being a protease itself) cleaves the Spike-protein through the remaining cleavage site on the S2 segment. That is exactly part of the CoV2 entry strategy. This second cleavage separates the two fusion proteins of S2, enabling them to fuse with the host cell membrane. Finally, in one last desperate attempt to drive off the virus, TMPRSS2 cleaves off the extracellular part of Ace2, causing it to be discarded.[26,27]

The membrane part of Ace2, still tightly bound to the RBD of CoV2, retracts back into the cell, dragging the virus with it. In this way, the virus is safely transported into the cell before is expelled, Ace2 receptor is destroyed and TMPRSS2 seems to be left intact.[28]

This is an incredible, almost science fiction, story of how a marvel of viral engineering engages two surface protease proteins in a choreographic sequence of savage bites and attempted escape maneuvers.

Lung Proteases – Ace2 and TMPRSS2

Our lungs express both proteases, TMPRSS2 and Ace2, on the same cells *in close proximity* to each other, which the virus uses to enter the cell. Many strains of influenza virus use TMPRSS2 as part of their infection strategy. The Spanish Flu, Hong Kong flu of 2009 and subsequent Bird flu outbreaks used it to great effect.[29]

Host epigenetics affect the levels of expression both TMPRSS2 and Ace2, with higher levels of these proteases increasing susceptibility to infection. Research has shown that people with a genetic variant that corresponds to a higher expression of TMPRSS2 in their lungs have a 2-fold higher risk of severe illness when exposed to the influenza virus.

Men have a higher susceptibility than women to influenza viruses and to CoV2. Not surprisingly, testosterone increases TMPRSS2 levels, explaining another layer of genetic susceptibility. Smoking likely also increases TMPRSS2 levels, making this a phenotypic effect. Inhaled cigarette smoke causes both normal (rs383510) and heightened expression gene (rs2070788) patients to increase TMPRSS2 levels. In essence, men with the rs2070788 gene who smoke are expected to suffer disproportionately more during this epidemic.[29]

The last big step to understanding COVID-19 is the role that Ace2 plays in lung health, and why losing Ace2 function during a CoV2 infection can be lethal. TMPRSS2 and Ace2 together predict susceptibility to infection, known as viral *tropism*. Ace2 degradation, which occurs during viral entry, predicts the host response to infection, known as *pathogenesis*.

Lung Ace2

There are two main types of cells lining the alveoli in the lungs. These cells are involved in secreting salt and water into the alveoli to keep them moist and they also secrete a vital protein complex called *surfactant*. Surfactant keeps the lungs flexible, making it easier to breath. Proteins in surfactant help with immune defense and reduce inflammation, essentially acting as frontline interferon and antibodies to disable viruses on arrival.[30]

Being an integral part of oxygen delivery, lung cells also receive the generalized RAS stress signal, AngII, through their AR1 receptors. AngII-mediated stress in these cells results in excessive fluid extravasation and inflammation in the delicate alveoli. This is how RAS stress causes chronic lung disease.

Ace2 is the protease tasked with cleaving AngII, thereby reducing the systemic inflammatory stress signal and preserving optimal lung function. Stressed lung cells increase expression of Ace2 enzymes to degrade the AngII signal when it is too strong. In essence, Ace2 protects the lungs by moderating the stress response to being overweight and sedentary.[31]

CELL ENTRY
CoV2 Meets Ace2

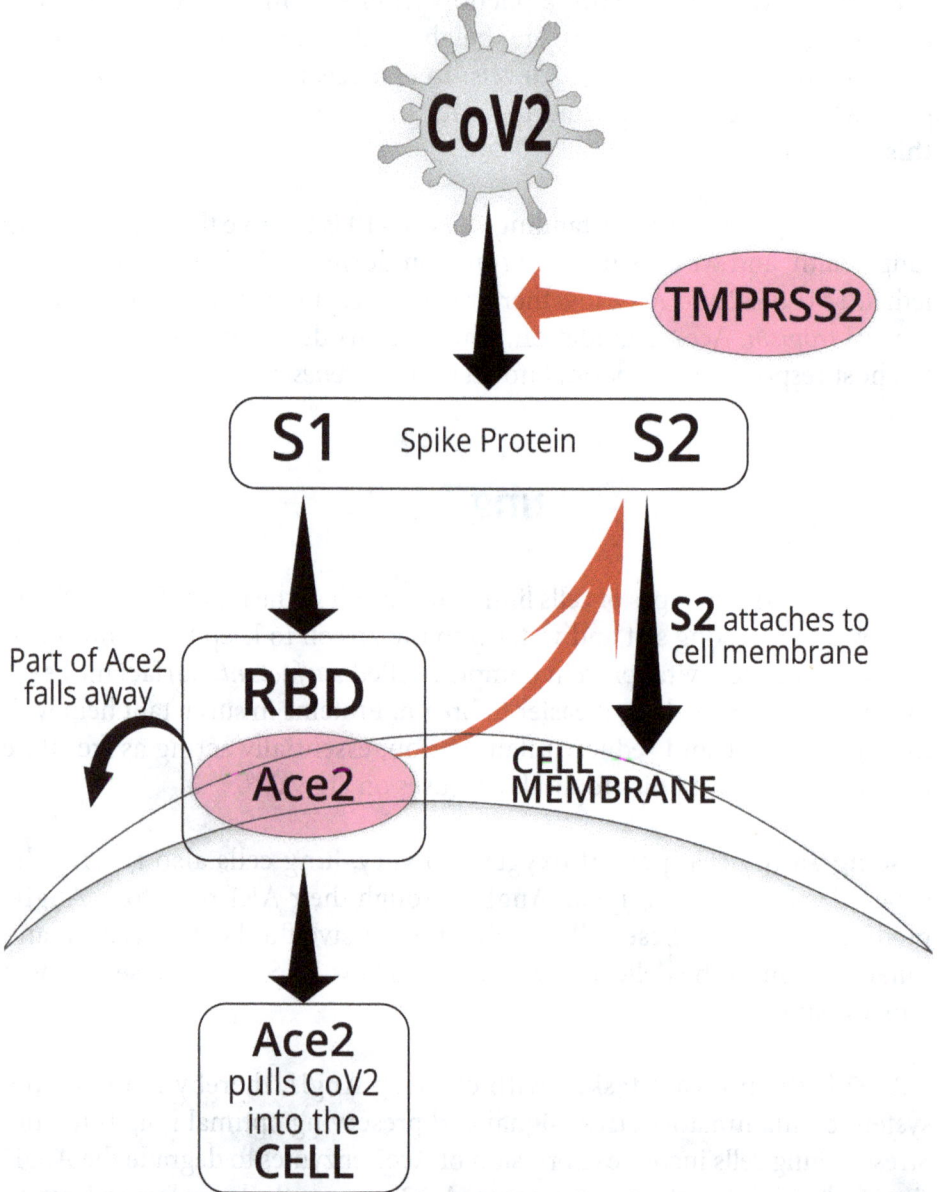

CoV2

TMPRSS2

S1 Spike Protein S2

S2 attaches to cell membrane

Part of Ace2 falls away

RBD

Ace2

CELL MEMBRANE

Ace2
pulls CoV2
into the
CELL

The frightening aspect of CoV2 is its targeted destruction of Ace2. In a young healthy population, this is not as much of a concern and may explain why they seem to be coping better with this infection. RAS-challenged metabolic syndrome patients, who make up a large portion of our middle-aged and older populations, will not fair nearly as well.[32]

The three new coronaviruses are deadly to diabetics and RAS stressed patients. Initial Covid-19 experience in Italy seems to confirm this observation. We have not seen this virus let loose on the North American population yet. I am terrified of what lies ahead. Covid-19 may be so selectively lethal that, to those affected, it may appear to be vindictive.

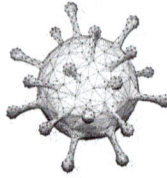

COVID-19 THE DISEASE

How It Started in Wuhan

The source of the first infection still remains unknown. In light of the stealthy onset of the disease, it is likely that the first transmission happened in November 2019. As we are witnessing in other countries, the virus spreads silently between people before emerging weeks later in clusters of cases.[33, 34]

Things started to go wrong in the first weeks of December 2019 in the city of Wuhan, in the central Hubei province of China. Wuhan is a large metropolitan city of 12 million people with an advanced infrastructure and economy. It is also the major rail transport hub of China, carrying millions of travellers over the Chinese New Year in January.

Initially, three people from the same family were admitted to hospital with fever, cough, malaise and shortness of breath. This would have brought back memories of SARS from 15 years earlier, even though SARS originated in Guangdong province south of Hubei. Chest x-rays and CT scans on the patients confirmed fluid in the lungs where there should have been air, something that could have been caused by a bacterial pneumonia or a viral pneumonitis. Blood tests confirmed normal or low white blood cell counts consistent with viral infection. When the patients did not respond to antibiotic treatment, a viral cause was suspected and the patients were isolated.

By the end of December 2019, it was announced that 27 cases of atypical pneumonia, 7 of them critically ill, had been identified in Wuhan. A local health alert was issued and the WHO was notified of the new outbreak on January 3, 2020.

Contact tracing revealed that these initial patients all had a close relationship with the Huanan Seafood Market, where live animals were sold. Most of the early patients were stall workers at the market and the animals sold included birds, bats, hedgehogs, marmots, pangolins, tiger frogs and snakes – all known coronavirus hosts.

At first, it was hoped that, as was the case with Bird flu, the virus would not spread *between* humans but only from animals to humans. If that were so, identifying the animal source and blocking further transfer would have stopped the outbreak relatively easily; however, person-to-person transmission of Covid-19 was confirmed when five people in a family, unrelated to the market, developed symptoms. The first local health alert was posted on December 31, 2019 and the now infamous Huanan Seafood Market was closed the very next day.

Wuhan has a strong and effective medical community. Fluid samples from the first patients were collected and a virus was isolated on January 7, 2020. It was identified and gene-sequenced on January 10. Samples were shared with other laboratories around the world, and the race was on.

We can only imagine the sense of terror and despair that gripped the virologists involved in these early days. Spouses would have been woken by distressed partners rushing to communicate with colleagues already at work in other parts of the world. A test to confirm the virus was developed on January 11.

This new CoV-Disease was listed on January 20, 2020 as a Notifiable Disease, in effect mandating reporting of all new cases. The city of Wuhan was essentially shut down on January 23 along with 15 other cities where cases were being reported. It took just 30 days to infect 30 provinces despite 1.4 billion people being isolated for 10 days over Chinese New Year. Almost 60 million people were confined to their homes for 50 days. Hospital bed numbers were increased from 2,000 to 50,000 and three new hospitals were built in just weeks. Forty thousand health care workers were mobilized.

The slow and quiet incubation time of this infection made it impossible to know what was happening in the population in those early days. Researchers started working on identifying cases, tracing transmission routes and calculating rates of spread. The R-0 was calculated to be anywhere from 1.4 to 6.47, indicating a mild spread rate at 1.4 to catastrophic at 6.47.

At the outset, authorities could only count people who self-identified as being sick without being able to confirm the disease through testing. Without an overall infection rate, it was impossible to calculate the percentage of patients who became very ill or died. Within 6 weeks of the first patient arriving in hospital, 9692 cases were confirmed. On January 31, China announced 15,238 suspected cases, with 213 deaths and 171 cures.

Infected patients were isolated and treated for ARDS with oxygen, mechanical ventilation and even oxygenation of blood outside their bodies, if required. Patients started to die as new patients presented in increasing numbers. There were likely many undiagnosed cases in the incubation phase and who knew how many infected patients would die in the days ahead. The numbers were changing daily and it was impossible to make accurate predictions.

The virus spread so quickly with new cases doubling every day or two that it was soon apparent that a citywide quarantine was required. Wuhan and other cities were put on quarantine on January 23. All public transport was shut down and roads in and out of the city were closed. Public places that attracted crowds such as restaurants and cinemas were closed. People were encouraged to wear masks in public. To many of us outside China, these measures seemed draconian at the time.

Unfortunately, the shutdown only occurred after many inhabitants had left Wuhan, either for the Chinese New Year or to escape the contagion. Compare that scenario to the single SARS patient who travelled to Hong Kong and infected 11 others at the start of the SARS epidemic.

It is important also to understand the implications of the term "confirmed cases". This test is used to identify viral RNA in a body fluid sample. The virus was only isolated and genetically typed o January 10, 2020. A test to identify it still had to be developed, produced, distributed put into use.

Testing for a respiratory-targeted virus starts with obtaining a throat swab from a sick patient. We know that this virus targets the lower respiratory tract, which accounts for the 25% false-negative test rate when sampling the upper respiratory tracts of infected patients. It is sobering to think that a quarter of those who are infected might test negative. It only took one patient to start this whole epidemic just a few months ago. So, any patient falsely identified as not being infected could restart the pandemic. We may need to self-isolate even with a negative test.

A general shutdown of movement was considered the only way to gain control in China. Hundreds of millions of people were confined in their homes for weeks. An anxious world awaits the results of the China's effort to contain the virus. Although their efforts at controlling spread seemed to be working, the virus had already spread to every continent before the end of February.

This viral outbreak is quite different from a nuclear power plant disaster, where leaking radioactive material spreads outwards from the source to contaminate the world. Radioactive spread must be contained at the source, and can only be achieved by the heroic efforts of those on site. A virus, on the other hand, spreads by its innate ability to replicate wherever it goes. This is not a localized situation with a ground zero located far away from us. *Each infected person is a ground zero.* We are all going to have to quarantine ourselves as strictly as the Chinese people have done if we are going to contain this. *We are all Wuhan now.*

China may yet be congratulated for the way in which it managed the initial outbreak. Certainly, we can learn from China as we all stare down CoV2. This is not the time for blame and acrimony. This is not the time for conspiracy theories that foster distrust and dissention.

The Spread of Covid-19

As the epidemic transitions into a pandemic and spreads around the world, it helps to understand that the numbers that we are given through the media are already historic and tend to under-report actual events.

Two important factors must be borne in mind. First, although Covid-19 has a 5-7day silent incubation period, it can become contagious during this time. Second, Covid-19 seems to have a R-0 of around 2.5 with a doubling time of five days. This will change as each country takes steps to reduce human contact through social distancing and isolation.[35,36,37]

Confirming cases requires a test that is not yet available in many countries. As such, authorities are unable to report the true incidence of new cases in their countries and we are unable to grasp the full extent of new infections.

With quarantine in effect, it may be difficult to determine spread through the quarantined population as they are essentially locked up at home. Additionally, we should assume that almost everyone confined with an infected patient would become infected.

The quandary facing China and other jurisdictions under quarantine is how long the lock-down should remain in force. Governments will have to weigh up the economic costs of a shutdown against the probability of reigniting the epidemic. Since identification and isolation of cases on an *ad hoc* basis has failed, there is no right answer to this dilemma. Returning society to normal after this is over is going to pose another set of challenges. China will likely be the advance guard, leading the way again.

Infected humans excrete this virus from every orifice. It is in our sputum, feces and urine. CoV2 is virulent enough to be spread by aerosol. Infected people breathing normally can spread the virus to others a few feet away, or possibly indirectly through air ducting systems. We must all be mindful that coronaviruses can survive outside of their hosts for hours, if not days.[38]

The Clinical Picture of Covid-19

Inhaled viruses are deposited in the lung of their new host. Alveolar epithelial cells and their backup white blood cells must defend 500 million alveoli with a combined surface area of $150m^2$ that is exposed to 12,000 liters of air every day. It is an intricate and well-controlled system. Too much defense will impair oxygen absorption, while too little can result in an overwhelming infection and death.

A week or two after infection with CoV2 the lung starts to mount a response. Interferons and cytokines set about destroying the virus and calling in help. As we noted above, inflammation causes blood vessels in the lung to become leaky and allow fluid extravasation.[39,40,41] Excess fluid in the lung alveoli hampers oxygen diffusion into the blood vessels on the other side of the alveolar membrane. Patients find it harder to breath, feel short of breath, and start to cough as their oxygen levels drop.[42]

Once the body is hypoxic with low blood oxygen, organs like the liver start emitting their ancient stress signal – angiotensinogen. This RAS signal causes salt and water retention, raises blood pressure and increases lung fluid. This is not a good time to increase lung fluid.

When this RAS signal threatens to overwhelm the lung its Ace2 proteins counter the message by breaking down the angiotensin proteins and converting them into anti-inflammatory signals. In this way, Ace2 improves survival.[43]

This is the key to understanding why Covid-19 can be deadly. After a heavy viral load in the lungs has ravaged the population of Ace2 proteins, there may not be enough Ace2 receptors left to quell the inflammatory RAS effect. Increasing fluid lung fluid further impairs oxygenation, which, in turn, increases angiotensinogen, leading to even more fluid retention. This sets up a classic feed-forward loop that can escalate rapidly.

COVID-19 RISK LIST

LOW RISK	HIGH RISK
Young (Less than 20 Years)	Old (Greater than 60 Years)
Female	Male
Blood Group O	Blood Group A
Non-Smoker	Smoker
Healthy Ideal Body Weight (BMI less than 25)	Metobolic Syndrome High Blood Pressure Heart Disease Diabetes (BMI greater than 30)
Exercises (Fit)	Sedentary Lifestyle (Unfit)

The best way to interrupt this stress loop is to raise blood oxygen levels. Oxygen is *critical* at this point. Just as masks and isolation are critical to prevent viral spread, oxygen is critical for survival once lung inflammation starts. The importance of oxygen is going to place a high demand on our ability to provide oxygen therapy in the months ahead.

Supplemental oxygen is required when the lungs are flooded with excess fluid, whatever the cause. We can boost our inhaled oxygen concentration from its natural level of 21% to 100%, if needed. Even at a 100% there may be insufficient uptake into the blood stream, as measured by the oxygen saturation of hemoglobin in the blood (0_2 saturation). Patients with persistent hypoxia despite 100% oxygen require intubation with a breathing tube placed directly into the trachea and mechanical (artificial) ventilation.

Artificial ventilation is also called positive pressure ventilation. An appropriate volume of oxygen is carefully blown through the endotracheal tube into the lung at a set rate and pressure. This is done in an intensive care or operating room setting and it really is *intensive care.*

Air pressure created by the ventilator to force oxygen into the patient also helps to literally push some of the lung fluid back into the blood vessels, while some of the extra fluid can be suctioned out of the lung via the endotracheal tube. Breathing for the patient also allows the diaphragm to rest, reducing its need for oxygen and sparing oxygen for the rest of the body. Labored breathing can consume as much as 20% of our oxygen.

Obviously, it is no fun to be intubated and ventilated so the patient is usually sedated with anesthetic medications and sedatives. The patient may even be paralyzed with a nerve-conduction blocking drug, especially if they are not oxygenating well. Paralysis can have a dramatic effect and is fully reversible.

While a patient is being ventilated with a presumed viral infection, the doctors need to decide whether to use antibiotic treatment. Although antibiotics will not have any effect on the virus, bacteria and even fungi can take advantage of the extra lung fluid and start opportunistic infections. If the patient has a history of chronic lung infections, antibiotics may be used early.

Failure to maintain blood oxygen saturation above 90% impairs the ability of the body to settle inflammation. This is when doctors might resort to a short course of high-dose steroids, to decrease inflammation just enough to improve oxygenation. Prolonged steroid might have been harmful during the SARS epidemic; therefore, if the patient does not respond, there may be no benefit in continuing steroids.

If lung inflammation does not settle and the patient can no longer be ventilated effectively, they will not survive. At this point, the doctors may resort to ECMO as a last-ditched treatment. ECMO stands for **e**xtra **c**orporeal **m**embrane **o**xygenation and involves putting the patient on a by-pass lung machine. During this procedure, the patient's heart keeps pumping blood through the oxygenating apparatus. This is distinct from heart-lung bypass used during open-heart surgery, where the heart is stopped.

During ECMO, a portion of the circulation is routed through a large tube placed in the femoral artery and run through a blood oxygenator which works like a lung. The oxygenated blood is returned back to the patient via the femoral vein.

ECMO is very expensive and intensive and is not widely available. Although ECMO does exist and may be effective sometimes, resource allocation will be a limiting factor. Unfortunately, reports from Italy this past week indicate that ECMO may not be effective in treating Covid-19 patients.

The heart and blood vessels also express Ace2 enzymes, making them highly susceptible to CoV2 entry and the resulting acute Ace2 depletion in those organs too. Loss of Ace2 increases oxidative stress, which has the catastrophic effect of un-coupling the nitric oxide producing proteins called *nitric oxide synthase* (NOS). Uncoupled NOS, instead, produces oxidized nitric oxide, called peroxynitrite, a highly reactive molecule that greatly accentuates oxidative stress.[44,45] Doctors may start using inhaled nitric oxide to help in these situations.

Uncoupled NOS is one of the major mechanisms accounting for cardiovascular disease. It seems to provide the mechanistic link between smoking and cardiovascular disease. Although NOS can be considered separately from the RAS system, the final common effect is mediated through oxidative stress in the heart. Combining RAS stress with NOS dysfunction is catastrophic and is seen when patients with metabolic syndrome and diabetes continue to smoke.

Peroxynitrite reduces blood flow to the heart muscle by constricting the coronary arteries, where nitric oxide would normally dilate them. The sudden increase in both AngII and peroxynitrite that occurs in severe Covid-19 infections causes the endothelial cells of the microcirculation in the heart to leak fluid, resulting in fluid collection in the heart muscle just as it occurs in the lung.

A heart that is low on oxygen and laboring to push blood through stiff wet lungs is less able to tolerate this additional oxidative stress in its own circulation. Hypoxia and interstitial fluid shifts are an anathema to hard working tissue such as cardiac muscle. It should be no surprise that patients in this situation experience sudden irreversible cardiac arrest. Unfortunately, sudden cardiac arrest may be a cause of death in predisposed Covid-19 patients.

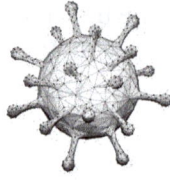

A LOOK AHEAD

A Looming Health Care Crisis

Treating Covid-19 patients in our hospitals opens another thorny issue around resource allocation. Our most valuable resource, our hospital staff, are going to be at risk of infection themselves. They may have to work long hours, increasing their own stress and the risk of dying. Fatigue increases the risk for errors with regard to self-protection, exposing workers to high doses of virus.

Tragically, healthcare workers died during the SARS epidemic of 2003. They died in China in January 2020 and will continue to do so in other countries. They could have stayed at home in self-imposed quarantine.

How will doctors and nurses in different countries respond to this threat? If they are pushed too hard and are not adequately supported with protective equipment and time off, then they will significantly increase their risk of getting sick. If some abandon their posts, their remaining colleagues will have to work harder, further increasing their risk of dying. This is another classic feed-forward loop.

Besides the increased personal risk assumed by health care workers, there is the added risk of spreading the virus both to other workers and to their families.

The relationship between the public and health care institutions will need to be nurtured by skilled and compassionate communicators. Families may not be allowed into hospitals to be at the bedside. They may not even be involved in decisions to offer or withdraw treatment. In fact, we may see a time soon when treatment may no longer be a right. This will be a time of great stress.

Reflections on This Evolving Pandemic

The hallmark of this coronavirus pandemic is its *stealth*. The rest of the world is beginning to understand what China was up against in those early days and why the country seemed to be unprepared and unable to manage the outbreak.

The human family will have to pool its efforts to contain Covid-19. We are all going to have to help. This is not the time to squabble. Although spread in the epicenter city of Wuhan seems to be contained, their efforts will have no impact on containment around the world. Newly infected countries have much to learn from Wuhan. There are already dozens of infection epicenters and each one is going to have to work equally as hard to contain spread in their countries.

Weighty political leadership is needed to stop travel and close schools and workplaces to contain this spread. History will judge the choices being made for us by our leaders over the next few weeks and months. Can we restrict movement of people sufficiently and long enough to contain this epidemic? Politicians must weigh pandemic risk against socioeconomic costs. There are optimists, pessimists and nihilists among us who reflect our collective emotions. We each choose who we follow. Ancient human emotions surface in the face of a plague.

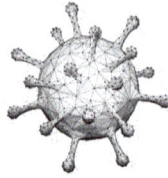

EPILOGUE

At the time of writing, three months have elapsed since the start of Covid-19. The number of new cases worldwide continues to double every 5 days. Total numbers now eclipse those in China, which are starting to decline. Under-reporting and ongoing scarcity of test kits make it impossible to determine the true incidence of new cases.

The Spanish Flu pandemic was caused by an H1N1 influenza virus mutation. Starting in January 1918, it infected 500 million people, almost 1/3 of the world's population before it ended in December 1920. The virus spread in two distinct waves, with a more virulent form showing up in the second wave. The source of the virus still remains open to speculation and many theories abound. It did not matter then and it does not matter now.

There have been two subsequent large influenza outbreaks since then. Asian flu in 1957 caused 2 million deaths and Hong Kong influenza in 1968 caused 1 million deaths, implying total infection rates of between 50 and 200 million people. We still have to cope with 5 million influenza infections every year with a mortality rate of about 0.1%, or 5000 people, despite mass influenza vaccination programs and cumulative herd immunity.

CoV2's silent spreading ability and 5-day doubling time, despite our best efforts, puts it in the same category as the Spanish flu. A third of the world's population may be infected before this is over in a year or two.

Based on spread patterns to date, the number of cases will increase ten-fold every month. By the end of December 2019 the total number was about 1000.

That number increased to 10,000 by the end of January, climbing to 100,000 at the end of February and by the end of March it might be up to 1 million.

With ongoing spread at this rate, the total number of recorded cases in the world will be almost ten million by the end of April 2020 and into the tens of millions as we go into the northern hemisphere summer. Spread must be contained before that point.

The ratio of infected people to confirmed cases is a major unknown factor. The incubation time from infection to symptoms is about 5 - 15 days, which is about two to four doubling cycles. It is likely that there are already 5 times as many undetected patients as there are newly diagnosed patients.

The only reliable statistics that we have for this pandemic so far are the number of deaths and number of patients who have recovered from a symptomatic illness. The three stages of the illness, incubation, symptomatic illness and pneumonitis may take as long as 28 days before the patient recovers or dies.

Since both are final outcomes and have a similar lag-time from the onset of infection, comparing the number of deaths to the number of recoveries may provide a realistic picture of Covid-19. A cursory look at the ratio of these numbers does not paint a rosy picture at all.

The combined total number of deaths and recoveries represents the total number of known patients who were sickened by Covid-19. If we then look at the death rate of that group of patients who can all be considered to have run the gauntlet of Covid-19, then we see that 20% of them died!

As the disease spreads and more of us become infected, we will be turning our attention to treatments, both to reduce the risk of developing pneumonitis and to help those who do, to survive.

Drugs that show promise will be rushed into production and distributed for clinical use. We will need to be careful. We will need to monitor and evaluate all new treatments, even as we are using them. We need to reflect on what an "FDA approval" means in the context of this crisis. In the context of Covid-19, an FDA approval will be permission to use a promising drug, at our own risk.

Our lives will forever be changed by the Pandemic of 2020. By understanding the moving parts and how they all fit together, we can build a collective consciousness around CoV2 that will help get us back to a new normal as soon as possible.

❧

REFERENCES

1. Morse SS, Mazet JA, Woolhouse M, et al. Prediction and prevention of the next pandemic zoonosis. *The Lancet*. 2012;380(9857):1956-1965.
2. Dallas TA, Carlson CJ, Poisot T. Testing predictability of disease outbreaks with a simple model of pathogen biogeography. *Royal Society Open Science*. 2019;6(11):190883.
3. Patel S, Rauf A, Khan H, Abu-Izneid T. Renin-angiotensin-aldosterone (RAAS): The ubiquitous system for homeostasis and pathologies. *Biomedicine & Pharmacotherapy*. 2017;94:317-325.
4. Yasue S, Masuzaki H, Okada S, et al. Adipose Tissue–Specific Regulation of Angiotensinogen in Obese Humans and Mice: Impact of Nutritional Status and Adipocyte Hypertrophy. *American Journal of Hypertension*. 2010;23(4):425-431.
5. Jia H. Pulmonary Angiotensin-Converting Enzyme 2 (ACE2) and Inflammatory Lung Disease: *SHOCK*. 2016;46(3):239-248.
6. Tikellis C, Bernardi S, Burns WC. Angiotensin-converting enzyme 2 is a key modulator of the renin–angiotensin system in cardiovascular and renal disease: *Current Opinion in Nephrology and Hypertension*. 2011;20(1):62-68.
7. Crackower MA, Sarao R, Oudit GY, et al. Angiotensin-converting enzyme 2 is an essential regulator of heart function. *Nature*. 2002;417(6891):822-828.
8. Guang C, Phillips RD, Jiang B, Milani F. Three key proteases – angiotensin-I-converting enzyme (ACE), ACE2 and renin – within and beyond the renin-angiotensin system. *Archives of Cardiovascular Diseases*. 2012;105(6-7):373-385.
9. de Wilde AH, Snijder EJ, Kikkert M, et al. Host Factors in Coronavirus Replication. *Current Topics in Microbiology and Immunology*. 2018;419:1-42.
10. Walter EJ, Hanna-Jumma S, Carraretto M, Forni L. The pathophysiological basis and consequences of fever. *Critical Care*. 2016;20(1)200.
11. Zhao J, Yang Y, et al. *Relationship between the ABO Blood Group and the COVID-19 Susceptibility*. Epidemiology; 2020. http://medrxiv.org/lookup/doi/10.1101/2020.03.11.20031096.
12. Fehr AR, Perlman S. Coronaviruses: An Overview of Their Replication and Pathogenesis. *Methods in Molecular Biology*. 2015;1282:1-23.
13. Gorbalenya AE, Baker SC, Baric RS, et al. *Severe Acute Respiratory Syndrome-Related Coronavirus: The Species and Its Viruses – a Statement of the Coronavirus Study Group*. Microbiology; 2020. http://biorxiv.org/lookup/doi/10.1101/2020.02.07.937862.

14. Li F. Receptor recognition and cross-species infections of SARS coronavirus. *Antiviral Research*. 2013;100(1):246-254.
15. Christian MD, Poutanen SM, Loutfy MR, et al. Severe Acute Respiratory Syndrome. *Clinical Infectious Diseases*. 2004;38(10):8.
16. Ge X-Y, Li J-L, Yang X-L, et al. Isolation and characterization of a bat SARS-like coronavirus that uses the ACE2 receptor. *Nature*. 2013;503(7477):535-538.
17. Stockman LJ, Bellamy R, Garner P. SARS: Systematic Review of Treatment Effects. *PLoS Medicine*. 2006;3(9):e343.
18. Al-Omari A, Rabaan AA, Salih S, et al. MERS coronavirus outbreak: Implications for emerging viral infections. *Diagnostic Microbiology and Infectious Disease*. 2019;93(3):265-285.
19. Song Z, Xu Y, Bao L, et al. From SARS to MERS, Thrusting Coronaviruses into the Spotlight. *Viruses*. 2019;11(1):59.
20. The Novel Coronavirus Pneumonia Emergency Response Epidemiology Team. The epidemiological characteristics of an outbreak of 2019 novel coronavirus diseases (COVID-19) in China. https://www.unboundmedicine.com/medline/citation/32064853/[The_epidemiological_characteristics_of_an_outbreak_of_2019_novel_coronavirus_diseases__COVID_19__in_China]_.
21. Menachery VD, Yount BL, Debbink K, et al. A SARS-like cluster of circulating bat coronaviruses shows potential for human emergence. *Nature Medicine*. 2015;21(12):1508-1513.
22. Kuhn JH, Li W, Choe H, et al. Angiotensin-converting enzyme 2: a functional receptor for SARS coronavirus. *Cellular and Molecular Life Sciences*. 2004;61(21):2738-2743.
23. Izaguirre G. The Proteolytic Regulation of Virus Cell Entry by Furin and Other Proprotein Convertases. *Viruses*. 2019;11(9):837.
24. Song W, Gui M, Wang X, Xiang Y. Cryo-EM structure of the SARS coronavirus spike glycoprotein in complex with its host cell receptor ACE2. *PLOS Pathogens*. 2018;14(8):e1007236.
25. Shulla A, Heald-Sargent T, Subramanya G, et al. Transmembrane Serine Protease Is Linked to the Severe Acute Respiratory Syndrome Coronavirus Receptor and Activates Virus Entry. *Journal of Virology*. 2011;85(2):873-882.
26. Iwata-Yoshikawa N, Okamura T, Shimizu Y, et al. TMPRSS2 Contributes to Virus Spread and Immunopathology in the Airways of Murine Models after Coronavirus Infection. *Journal of Virology*. 2019;93(6):e01815-18.
27. Yan R, Zhang Y, Li Y, et al. Structural basis for the recognition of the SARS-CoV-2 by full-length human ACE2. *Science*. March 2020:eabb2762.

28. Belouzard S, Chu VC, Whittaker GR. Activation of the SARS coronavirus spike protein via sequential proteolytic cleavage at two distinct sites. *Proceedings of the National Academy of Sciences.* 2009;106(14):5871-5876.

29. Cheng Z, Zhou J, To KK-W, et al. Identification of TMPRSS2 as a Susceptibility Gene or Severe 2009 Pandemic A(H1N1) Influenza and A(H7N9) Influenza. *Journal of Infectious Diseases.* 2015;212(8):1214-1221.

30. Guillot L, Nathan N, Tabary O, et al. Alveolar epithelial cells: Master regulators of lung homeostasis. *The International Journal of Biochemistry & Cell Biology.* 2013;45(11):2568-2573.

31. Imai Y, Kuba K, Rao S, et al. Angiotensin-converting enzyme 2 protects from severe acute lung failure. *Nature.* 2005;436(7047):112-116.

32. Kuba K, Imai Y, Rao S, et al. A crucial role of angiotensin converting enzyme 2 (ACE2) in SARS coronavirus–induced lung injury. *Nature Medicine.* 2005;11(8):875-879.

33. Li Q, Guan X, Wu P, et al. Early Transmission Dynamics in Wuhan, China, of Novel Coronavirus–Infected Pneumonia. *New England Journal of Medicine.* 2020;382(13):1199-1207.

34. Report of the WHO-China Joint Mission on Coronavirus Disease 2019 (COVID-19). https://www.who.int/publications-detail/report-of-the-who-china-joint-mission-on-coronavirus-disease-2019-(covid-19).

35. Lauer SA, Grantz KH, Bi Q, et al. The Incubation Period of Coronavirus Disease 2019 (COVID-19) From Publicly Reported Confirmed Cases: Estimation and Application[published online ahead of print, 2020 Mar 10]. *Annals of Internal Medicine.* 2020;M20-0504.

36. Liu Y, Gayle AA, Wilder-Smith A, Rocklöv J. The reproductive number of COVID-19 is higher compared to SARS coronavirus. *Journal of Travel Medicine.* 2020; 27(2):taaa021.

37. Backer JA, Klinkenberg D, Wallinga J. Incubation period of 2019 novel coronavirus (2019-nCoV) infections among travellers from Wuhan, China, 20–28 January 2020. *Eurosurveillance.* 2020;25(5):200062.

38. Lai C-C, Shih T-P, Ko W-C, et al. Severe acute respiratory syndrome coronavirus 2 (SARS-CoV-2) and coronavirus disease-2019 (COVID-19): The epidemic and the challenges. *International Journal of Antimicrobial Agents.* 2020;55(3):105924.

39. Wang D, Hu B, Hu C, et al. Clinical Characteristics of 138 Hospitalized Patients With 2019 Novel Coronavirus–Infected Pneumonia in Wuhan, China [published online ahead of print, 2020 Feb7]. *JAMA.* 2020;e201585.

40. Yang X, Yu Y, Xu J, et al. Clinical course and outcomes of critically ill patients with SARS-CoV-2 pneumonia in Wuhan, China: a single-centered, retrospective, observational study [published online ahead of print, 2020 Feb 24] [published correction appears in Lancet Respir Med. 2020 Feb 28;:]. The Lancet Respiratory Medicine. 2020;S2213-2600(20)30079-5.

41. Guan W, Ni Z, Hu Y, et al. Clinical Characteristics of Coronavirus Disease 2019 in China[published online ahead of print, 2020 Feb 28]. *New England Journal of Medicine.* 2020.

42. Zhu N, Zhang D, Wang W, et al. A Novel Coronavirus from Patients with Pneumonia in China, 2019. *New England Journal of Medicine.* 2020;382(8):727-733.

43. Nagata N, Iwata N, Hasegawa H, et al. Mouse-Passaged Severe Acute Respiratory Syndrome-Associated Coronavirus Leads to Lethal Pulmonary Edema and Diffuse Alveolar Damage in Adult but Not Young Mice. *The American Journal of Pathology.* 2008;172(6):1625-1637.

44. Kuba K, Imai Y, Penninger JM. Multiple Functions of Angiotensin-Converting Enzyme 2 and Its Relevance in Cardiovascular Diseases. *Circulation Journal.* 2013;77(2):301-308.

45. Oudit GY, Crackower MA, Backx PH, et al. The Role of ACE2 in Cardiovascular Physiology. *Trends in Cardiovascular Medicine.* 2003;13(3):93-101.

ACKNOWLEDGMENTS

Nadine Gordon
My friend and researcher, 'The Dogged Researcher' who has responded to hundreds of "get me a review paper on …." texts and has tirelessly tracked down thousands of scientific papers for me, any day of the week, for over a decade.

Rob Bradizza
My editor, and still my friend, who neglected his family to jump into this project early enough in my writing to make his work quite onerous.

Chris Miner
My friend and photographer, who not only made me look presentable, but also indulged my whim with other photo concepts for this project.

Lynne McMullan
My friend and designer, who worked on numerous cover designs and layout options until I was content.

ABOUT THE AUTHOR

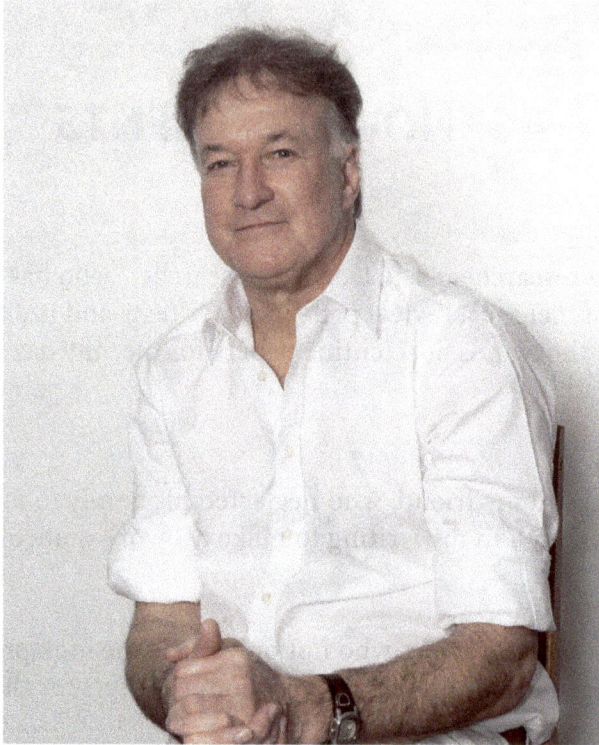

Dr. Richard Henry

I am an Assistant Professor at Queen's University in Canada. I trained here in Anesthesiology and stayed these past 30 years, teaching students and residents and learning from my colleagues and patients. My hospital work is mainly in the operating room. My specialized clinical skills are in neonatal anesthesia and chronic pain.

I am a third generation 'white' South African. I thrived in Africa, but grieved under apartheid. Although I treasure my education, none of us will forget the emotional turmoil we all felt working in segregated health care. Even the mortuary was racially divided.

It was under that deluge of social diseases that I gradually developed a habit of trying to understand health in its full context. It's been 35 years since I was welcomed by Canada. I like to think that while South Africa gave me my grit, Canada nurtured my joy of being a doctor and an inquisitive researcher.

My research for the past twenty years has been in chronic pain, which is still considered a sensory nerve system disorder. Following that logic, sensory-directed drugs such as opiates, anti-depressants and anti-epileptics remain in use. I came to believe that there had to a more valid explanation for chronic pain, and set out to find it.

My journey brought me to the realization that chronic pain is just another manifestation in the spectrum of our modern diseases, all with the same underlying mechanisms. The answer seems to be in the way that humans have *changed epigenetically.* I embarked on a book on epigenetics and modern disease, but put it aside when I came to the shocking realization in late January 2020 that Covid-19 was going to challenge this maladapted state.

For most of my time in Canada, I have made Kingston, Ontario my home. It is a gentle town at the end of the Great Lakes, just as Lake Ontario narrows to become the St. Lawrence River. Queen's University and my home are a short, contemplative, walk apart along the water's edge. I have four Canadian-born adult children who, too, enjoy the opportunities offered by a wonderfully inclusive and cooperative society.

I am a father, a son and a brother, a friend, colleague, scholar and, yes, a doctor. I am grateful for what Canada has afforded me, and remain mindful of the guiding wisdoms that surrounded me at home in my early life.

South Africans have a few meanings for 'now', each of them with varying degrees of urgency. There's 'now!' as in 'this moment'. Then there's 'just now', meaning 'in a while' an artfully vague answer you give your nagging child. 'Now-now' has nothing to do with time, it's a soothing comment to calm things down. And then there's 'right now!', a 'now' with urgency and immediacy. In South Africa we might use 'now' like this: "We *must* all work together to fight this virus, *right now!*"

This is our moment, our call to serve for the greater good. It is time to drop differences and understand the urgency of working together as one human family, one human species, against a common threat. We have the expertise to drive out this virus. If we share our knowledge and skills, working from a common playbook, we *can* get this done sooner than 'just now'.

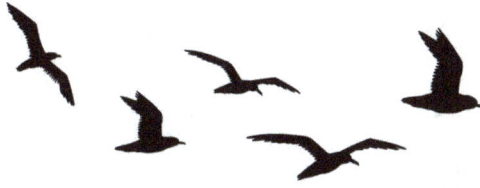

IN SPIRIT

I leave you with a short excerpt that I extracted from the book, Jonathan Livingston Seagull. I typed it out in 1975 while in boarding school and have had it on my desk since. I re-gift it to you from this timeless work by Richard Bach.

Most gulls don't bother to learn more than the simplest facts of flight – how to get from shore to food and back again. It's all so pointless, there's so much to learn.

It was pretty just to stop thinking; but one who has touched excellence in his learning has no need of that kind of promise.

He was alive, trembling ever so slightly with delight, proud that his fear was under control. His thought was triumph. How much more there is now to living! Instead of our drab slogging there's a reason to life! We can lift ourselves out of ignorance, we can find ourselves as creatures of excellence and intelligence and skill. We can be free!

…in the very times when every other gull stood on the ground, knowing nothing but mist and rain, he learned to ride the high winds far inland, to dine there on delicate insects.
Jonathan Seagull discovered that boredom and fear and anger are the reasons that a gull's life is so short.

Excerpts from
Jonathan Livingston Seagull
by Richard Bach

www.ingramcontent.com/pod-product-compliance
Lightning Source LLC
Chambersburg PA
CBHW061612220326
41598CB00024BC/3556